Hot Topics
for MRCGP
and
General Practitioners

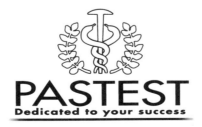

Hot Topics for MRCGP and General Practitioners

Louise R Newson
BSc (Hons) MBChB (Hons) MRCP MRCGP
GP Principal
Kenilworth
Warwickshire

Ash M Patel
MBChB MRCGP DRCOG DFFP
GP Principal
Bramhall
Cheshire

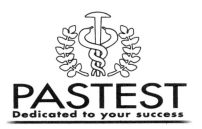

© 2001 PASTEST Ltd
Egerton Court
Parkgate Estate
Knutsford
Cheshire
WA16 8DX

Telephone: 01565 752000

All rights reserved. No part of this publication may be reproduced, stored in a retrieval system, or transmitted, in any form or by any means, electronic, mechanical, photocopying, recording or otherwise without the prior permission of the copyright owner.

First published 2001

ISBN 1 901198 81 2

A catalogue record for this book is available from the British Library.

The information contained within this book was obtained by the authors from reliable sources. However, while every effort has been made to ensure its accuracy, no responsibilty for loss, damage or injury occasioned to any person acting or refraining from action as a result of information contained herein can be accepted by the publishers or authors.

PasTest Revision Books and Intensive Courses

PasTest has been established in the field of postgraduate medical education since 1972, providing revision books and intensive study courses for doctors preparing for their professional examinations.

Books and courses are available for the following specialties:

MRCGP, MRCP Part 1 and 2, MRCPCH Part 1 and 2, MRCPsych, MRCS, MRCOG, DRCOG, DCH, FRCA, PLAB.

For further details contact:

PasTest, Freepost, Knutsford, Cheshire WA16 7BR
Tel: 01565 752000   Fax: 01565 650264
www.pastest.co.uk   enquiries@pastest.co.uk

Text prepared by Breeze Ltd, Manchester.
Printed and bound by Bell and Bain Ltd, Glasgow.

CONTENTS

Foreword	viii
Introduction	ix
Why bother with Hot Topics?	x
Useful reading material	xii

Chapter 1: Chronic Diseases — 1

Hypertension
Coronary Heart Disease
The Coronary Heart Disease National Service Framework
Heart failure
Atrial fibrillation
Stroke
Diabetes mellitus
Osteoporosis

Chapter 2: Respiratory Diseases — 32

Asthma
Chronic obstructive airways disease
Smoking cessation
Influenza

Chapter 3: Obesity — 45

Chapter 4: Psychiatry — 48

Mental Health National Service Framework
Depression
Post-natal depression
Schizophrenia
The new anti-psychotic drugs
Eating disorders
Alcohol
Drugs
Counselling

Chapter 5: The Elderly — 74

The 'grey' army
Implications for healthcare
Implications for society
Dementia

Contents

Chapter 6: Obstetrics & Gynaecology   **97**
Combined oral contraceptive pill
Emergency contraception
Teenagers and sexual health
Chlamydia
Hormone replacement therapy

Chapter 7: Paediatrics   **111**
Childhood Vaccinations
Sudden infant death syndrome

Chapter 8: Cancer   **114**
NHS Cancer Plan
Prostate cancer

Chapter 9: Antibiotics   **122**
Antibiotic resistance
Antibiotics and acute otitis media
Sore throat

Chapter 10: Clinical Governance   **129**

Chapter 11: Revalidation   **135**
Practice and personal development plans
Practice professional developments plans (PPDPs)

Chapter 12: The Future of General Practice   **146**
The NHS Plan
Rationing
Primary care groups
Personal medical services (PMS) pilots
Out of hours care and 24 hour responsibility
NHS Direct
Walk-in centres
Nurse practitioners
Outreach clinics
Practice formulary
Computer-generated repeat prescriptions
Post-'Shipman'

Contents

Chapter 13: Medicine & the Internet   **177**

Chapter 14: Alternative medicine   **180**

Chapter 15: Medico-legal issues and guidelines   **183**
GMC
Complaints
Confidentiality
Consent
Medical negligence
Guidelines

Chapter 16: Advance Directives   **195**
End Of Life decisions

Chapter 17: Miscellaneous topics   **201**
Refugees
Recent ethical advances

Chapter 18: The Consultation   **208**
The Doctor-Patient Partnership
Consultation Models

Appendices   **220**
Glossary
Journals referenced in this book

Index   **223**

vii

FOREWORD

I am delighted to recommend this excellent book that has been written by two recently successful MRCGP candidates. The MRCGP examination requires a breadth of current knowledge, not only clinical but also the wider context of primary care. It is difficult to bring together all of the relevant information during a busy revision period yet success depends on achieving this. Louise Newson and Ash Patel are to be congratulated on their collection of essential and up-to-date information which will be invaluable not only to the examination candidate but also to their trainer. Even examiners will find it useful!

John Sandars MSc FRCGP MRCP
Examiner MRCGP Examination

ACKNOWLEDGEMENTS

We would like to thank our families, especially Paul and Priti, for all their patience, support and tolerance over the past few months.

We would also like to thank John Sandars for all his advice and encouragement in developing this book.

Finally, we thank the PasTest Publishing Department, as without their help and guidance, we would have never been able to create this book.

INTRODUCTION

The MRCGP exam seems like a long way off at the beginning of the Registrar year, but unfortunately it soon comes round! The amount of information required to work as a General Practitioner and to pass the exam can appear to be completely daunting and overwhelming.

When we were both preparing for the MRCGP exam in Summer 2000 we were disappointed to find a relative paucity of books and courses to help with 'hot topic' revision. Numerous laborious hours were spent trawling through and summarising back issues of the BMJ and BJGP by ourselves and with other members of our VTS group, hoping it would help with our revision but we found it quite a fruitless exercise. It is also sometimes difficult to prioritise and become familiar with the more important, well-researched papers on a topic.

This book has been designed to help you improve your breadth and depth of knowledge of various important clinical and non-clinical subjects. Medicine is a dynamic specialty and information is constantly being updated and theories altered as more research is performed and attitudes of both doctors and patients change.

It is impossible to predict topics for future exams successfully and for that reason the subjects covered in this book will be as relevant as possible to present and future general practice. This book is not meant to be a comprehensive revision course for the exam; it is written to provide some guidance and ideas upon which to base your revision. It will also hopefully save you some time by reducing the need for reading and summarising all the journals.

Each of the hot topics are presented as a broad overview with reference to recent literature. References, useful reading material and relevant web sites are also included for each topic.

We have therefore written this book to try to help and direct candidates with some of their revision. The reviews of various key 'hot topics' will be important for both the exam and also future careers in General Practice. The book will also be very useful for established GPs who would like a review of the current literature on a wide variety of topics.

WHY BOTHER WITH HOT TOPICS?

There are questions in Paper 1 (the written paper) specifically designed to test candidates' knowledge and interpretation of general practice literature. Candidates are expected to be familiar with items in the medical literature which have influenced current thinking in general practice. Paper 2 (the MCQs) has questions based on articles and reviews printed over the last eighteen months. The viva also concentrates on topics that require an awareness of the recent literature.

In addition, good GPs use evidence-based medicine as a starting point and are able to apply it to meet the needs and circumstances of an individual patient, and as a joint decision with the patient. A 'patient-centred' approach is a highly desirable quality for the MRCGP exam and for future practice.

MYTHS ABOUT HOT TOPICS FOR THE EXAM

You need to know everything
Although the amount of information you are expected to know may feel insurmountable, it is important to remember that it is impossible to know everything, the examiners certainly don't! There is no shame and indeed much credit in knowing your own and your professional limitations. Too much pride or arrogance can actually be off-putting to the examiners.

You need to be able to quote papers to pass the exam
Candidates are not expected to be able to quote individual references of articles. It is more important, for example, to know that there are many papers with different results regarding the treatment of sore throats with antibiotics rather than to know only one paper and its design faults in detail.

If you know a key paper was printed recently in the BMJ, for example, then it is worth stating. However, it is worse to misquote a reference or quote a reference in the wrong context than to not quote at all! The college states that inaccurate or incomplete references will not be penalised but misleading ones will.

Hot Topics are the most important part of revision for the exam
There has recently been more emphasis placed on candidates' awareness of current issues for the exam, especially as evidence-based medicine is becoming a very important part of clinical practice.

Why Bother With Hot Topics?

However, the examiners are actually more interested in ensuring that candidates are broad-minded, patient-centred and can consider problems in general practice from many different perspectives and be able to think about social, ethical, political and cultural factors. It is the application of any knowledge obtained rather than the knowledge itself which is important for both the exam and working in general practice.

Although 3 1/2 hours seems a long time for the written paper, the exam passes quickly with very little spare time. If candidates spend too much time on hot topics or current literature in their answers this may be detrimental because it leaves less time to spend on other very relevant issues. For example, when considering an answer about the optimal management of a newly diagnosed diabetic patient, the impact this diagnosis may have on both the patient and their family is equally as important as discussing various trials regarding target glycosylated haemoglobin levels.

USEFUL READING MATERIAL FOR 'HOT TOPICS' REVISION

There are a large number of revision books for the exam and a huge number of books about general practice. Your trainer and VTS scheme will be able to advise you about these.

It is generally advised that candidates should be up-to-date with the past eighteen months of the literature. However, it is worth bearing in mind that there are many older studies which still influence General Practice. The main journals to read are the *British Medical Journal* and the *British Journal of General Practice*, as exam questions are usually set from these and also they are the journals that examiners usually read! *Drugs and Therapeutics Bulletin* is a useful journal as it provides unbiased reviews. The new Clinical Evidence book, produced every six months by the BMJ is a useful reference source for evidence-based medicine.

The free weekly newspapers *GP*, *Pulse* and *Doctor* have very useful relevant discussion material, both clinical and non-clinical. *Update* also produces some very relevant articles and includes Self-Assessment exercises every month, which consist of MCQs, Modified Essay Questions, Short Answer Questions and a Critical Reading Exercise. These can be very useful to discuss with your trainer or in your study groups.

It is preferable to try to read some journals on a regular basis rather than trying to cram everything in the month before the exam. This not only makes last minute revision less stressful but it also means that some of the knowledge can be used during your clinical practice.

KEY POINTS

Do not panic!
You do not have to know everything
Try to read journals regularly
Use evidence-based medicine in your practice

USEFUL JOURNALS/PUBLICATIONS

British Medical Journal (BMJ)
British Journal of General Practice (BJGP)
Evidence-based Medicine
GP/Doctor/Pulse
Update
Drugs and Therapeutics Bulletin

CHAPTER 1: CHRONIC DISEASES

HYPERTENSION

Hypertension has been defined by the World Health Organisation (in 1993) as the blood pressure above which intervention has been shown to reduce risk. Hypertension is a very common but poorly managed condition. 50% of hypertensives are undetected, 50% of those detected are not treated and 50% of those treated are not adequately controlled.

How much should BP be lowered by?
A very large randomised controlled trial, the Hypertension Optimal Treatment Trial (HOT) looked at outcomes in terms of major cardiovascular disease (CVD) events *(Lancet 1998;351:1755-62)*. The BHS guidelines (see below) are based on this study. This showed that the lowest incidence of CVD events occurred at a mean diastolic blood pressure of 82.6 mmHg and the lowest CVD mortality at 86.5 mmHg. Even lower diastolic blood pressure was found beneficial in diabetics (optimal 80 mmHg).

The HOT study is the only study that has set out to evaluate optimal target BP levels and they reported an optimal pressure of 139/83 mmHg. This study also showed a 15% reduction in major CVD events and a 36% reduction in non-fatal MI with patients on aspirin. The benefit of aspirin for primary prevention had been controversial before this study.

British Hypertension Society (BHS) Guidelines *(BMJ 1999;319:630)*
These are evidence-based guidelines written largely by professors which aim to present the best currently available evidence on hypertension management. They recommend starting treatment on the basis of risk rather than blood pressure for patients with borderline hypertension.

Important points
- All adults should have their BP checked every five years, or every year if borderline
- All patients should receive non-pharmacological advice
- Initiate treatment if SBP >160 or DBP >100
- Consider treatment in borderline patients if target organ damage / diabetes / 10 year coronary risk >15%
- Choice of drug should be tailored to patient (e.g. ACEI for LVF, β-blockers for IHD)
- Aspirin should be considered if 10 year CVD risk >15%

Chronic Diseases

- Statins should be considered if 10 year CVD risk >30%
- Drug treatment is of proven value until age 80 years, over this decision to treat should be based on biological age

NB. 10 year coronary heart disease risk is estimated by using the risk chart issued by the Joint British Societies in their recommendations for coronary heart disease prevention *(Heart 1998;119:329–35)*.

Good points of guidelines
They are clear, concise and based on good evidence. They aim to address the incomplete detection, treatment and control of hypertension prevalent across all sections of the community. The emphasis on the assessment and reduction of cardiovascular **risk** rather than just the maintenance of an optimal blood pressure is to be welcomed.

Problems with these guidelines
Some of the treatment recommendations are based on consensus rather than evidence.

The resource implications are huge for GPs as the guidelines will result in a far greater proportion of patients needing treatment, monitoring and close follow-up.

It has been estimated that an average GP would have 272 patients aged under 75 years who would be eligible for treatment, which could mean a potential extra four hours of work a week to devote to their ongoing management!

There is no reference to patient preferences. Why choose a 10 year risk threshold of 15%? This means that over ten years, 19 out of 20 patients taking treatment will derive no benefit from it.

What are the risk tables?
They are based on the Framingham data, which came from a 10 year follow-up of 5000 patients. The risk equations from the Framingham data have been shown to be reasonably accurate when applied to other populations in northern Europe and USA – they have been criticised for not including other cardiovascular risk factors (such as family history, sedentary lifestyle and obesity). There are three main tables, The New Zealand, Sheffield and Joint British Societies. These take absolute rather than relative risk into consideration, which is far more relevant to individual patients.

Chronic Diseases

How do the different risk tables compare?

Both the Joint British Societies chart and the Sheffield table are compatible with UK guidelines. However, a study in primary care found that although the Sheffield table correctly identified slightly more people who were at high risk compared with the Joint British Societies chart, it also falsely labelled more low risk people as being at high risk. Overall this study concluded that the Joint British Societies chart has the best balance of accuracy *(Heart 2001;85:37–43)*.

How easy is it to measure cardiovascular risk for patients?

Accurate estimation of cardiovascular risk without the use of explicit risk charts or computer-based clinical decision support systems is not easy. Health professionals find it difficult to assimilate multiple risk factors into an accurate assessment of cardiovascular risk *(BMJ 2000;320:686–90)*.

What are the disadvantages of using the risk tables?

They can only be used for primary prevention. They do not apply to people with familial hyperlipidaemia as these patients are high risk. Ethnic minorities are not mentioned. Sections of the ethnic community, particularly Afro-Caribbeans and South Asians, are at greatly increased risk of end organ damage owing to hypertension. They also exhibit an increased incidence of concomitant cardiovascular risk factors such as diabetes and obesity. They also under-estimate the risk if there is a strong family history of coronary heart disease at a younger age. In addition, no allowances are made for heaviness of smoking or socio-economic status in the risk calculations.

How can risk clearly be given to patients?

Results of a study from a surgery in London has shown that patient decisions regarding medication are strongly affected by the way information is explained to them *(BJGP 2001;51:276–9)*. A questionnaire was sent to patients which asked their likelihood of accepting treatment for a chronic condition on the basis of relative risk reduction, absolute risk reduction, number needed to treat and personal probability of benefit. The results varied from 44% stating they would accept treatment with a personal probability of benefit model, to 92% stating they would accept treatment using a relative risk reduction model. This could therefore mean that the presentation of a risk statistic in 'everyday language' to ensure full comprehension may result in a proportion of patients refusing beneficial treatment.

What should we use to measure blood pressure?
In Sweden and the Netherlands the use of mercury is no longer permitted in hospitals. In the United Kingdom the move to ban mercury has not been received with enthusiasm because we do not have an accurate alternative to the mercury sphygmomanometer *(BMJ 2000;320:815)*. However, aneroid devices can be extremely inaccurate and automated devices vary enormously.

Are patients being over-treated?
An old study by Fry in 1979 demonstrated that 1 in 3 patients with hypertension became normotensive with time. This has been confirmed more recently in a study that found 20% of well controlled hypertensives could have their medication controlled without problems *(BJGP 1999;49:977--80)*. The overall conclusion regarding treatment choice is that it is the level of blood pressure that counts, not the drug used to treat it. It is sensible to prescribe medication that is most likely to suit your patient's past medical history and probably more important to choose a medication that is less likely to cause side-effects so improving compliance.

 USEFUL WEBSITES

www.hyp.ac.uk/bhs – British Hypertension Society (Includes copies of CVD risk charts)
www.bmj.com – British Medical Journal
www.bhf.org.uk – British Heart Foundation

ROUTINE INVESTIGATIONS FOR HYPERTENSION

- Urine dipstix for blood/protein
- Urea and creatinine
- Blood glucose
- Serum total:LDL cholesterol ratio
- 12 lead ECG

SUMMARY POINTS FOR HYPERTENSION

- Hypertension is underdiagnosed
- BHS guidelines have huge resource implications
- Familiarise yourself with risk tables
- Consider statins and aspirin
- BP targets are lower for diabetics

Chronic Diseases

CORONARY HEART DISEASE

The prevention of coronary heart disease (CHD) is one of the most important tasks for general practice. CHD remains the principal cause of death in the UK and a fifth of these deaths occur below retirement age. The main risk factors are smoking, hypertension, hypercholesterolaemia, diabetes and obesity.

Joint British recommendations on prevention of Coronary Heart Disease
These evidence-based guidelines were written by the British Cardiac and Hypertension Societies and the British Hyperlipidaemia and Diabetic Associations *(Heart 1998;80(suppl 2):S1-29, summary in BMJ 2000; 320:705)*. They recommend that priority should be given to patients at high absolute risk of coronary heart disease over a specified period, rather than an undue emphasis on an individual risk factor. They therefore follow the same principle as the British Hypertension Guidelines. The guidelines are simple to follow and realistic.

The medical priority is to focus on those who are at highest risk of CHD. The first priority is secondary prevention for patients with established CHD and the second priority is primary prevention for people at high risk of developing CHD; they are those people with an absolute CHD risk ≥15% over 10 years, as calculated using the Joint British Societies coronary risk prediction charts. The charts use information on age, gender, lipid profile and blood pressure to calculate a patient's risk. It is suggested (see over) that the people at a higher cardiovascular risk should start drug therapy but this is probably over ambitious given the current financial state of the NHS!

The implementation of this strategy is a major challenge for primary health care but it obviously links with the National Service Framework for Coronary Heart Disease (see page 10).

Chronic Diseases

The main points of these guidelines are:

Lifestyle targets for all patients	Stopping smoking; diet; exercise; moderate alcohol
Targets for other risk factors	BP <140/85 Total cholesterol <5.0 mmol/l
Diabetic patients	BP <130/80 HbA_{1C} <7%
Cardioprotective drugs	Aspirin for all patients with CVD and patients >50 years with controlled hypertension beta-blockers for at least 3 years post MI Statins if required ACE inhibitors for patients with heart failure or reduced ejection fraction (<40%) Warfarin for patients at risk of systemic embolism
Screening for first degree relatives	Of patients with premature CHD (men <55 years and women <65 years)

Risk factors for CHD
Health care professionals tend to over-emphasise the benefits of medication (e.g. statins) and neglect lifestyle factors (e.g. smoking, diet).

Improvements in risk factors and treatment have been shown to be associated with reductions in CHD in a large epidemiological study by the World Health Organisation. This study, MONICA, monitored 100,000 men and women aged 35–64 years from 21 countries over 10 years *(Lancet 2000; 355:668–9)*. However, the results were not as impressive as had been hoped. The most effective intervention was to stop smoking, which results in a 50% risk reduction over two years.

What are the benefits of lowering cholesterol?
There is overwhelming evidence that statins are highly beneficial in the secondary prevention of CHD. There are four large key trials regarding statin use and coronary heart disease:
* 4S – large randomised controlled trial of secondary prevention in patients with CHD and raised cholesterol *(Lancet 1994;344:1383–89)*

Chronic Diseases

- CARE – large trial of secondary prevention in patients with normal cholesterol post MI *(NEMJ 1996;335:1001–9)*
- LIPID – randomised controlled trial similar to CARE but with higher patient numbers *(NEMJ 1998; 339:1349–57)*
- WOSCOPS – randomised controlled trial of primary prevention in middle-aged men with raised cholesterol *(NEMJ 1995;333:1301–7)*

There is no longer any doubt that treatment benefits those who are at substantial coronary risk. An updated meta-analysis *(BMJ 2000; 321:96–8)* shows that drugs which lower lipid concentrations prevent nearly one-third of myocardial infarctions and coronary deaths. Yet many people who could substantially benefit from statins are not getting them, perhaps due to a lack of understanding by physicians or to poor organisation *(BMJ 2000;321:971–2)*. Recent data has shown that less than 33% of patients with a history of cardiovascular disease, and only 3% of people with a 10 year risk of coronary heart disease of ≥ 30%, are currently receiving lipid-lowering drugs, which is clearly inadequate *(BMJ 2000;321:1322–5)*. Treating all patients with a 10 year CHD risk of ≥ 15% would effectively mean statin treatment for about a quarter of the UK adult population – which is clearly not achievable with current NHS funding!

The NNT (number needed to treat) with statins for secondary prevention of death over 5 years is 16, i.e. 16 patients have to take a statin for 5 years to prevent one death. NNT for primary prevention is 69.

In addition, a recent study has shown that patients taking statins may also reduce their risk of developing Alzheimer's disease! *(Arch Neuro 2000;57:1439–43)*. This study reported that patients receiving lovastatin or pravastatin (but not simvastatin) had a 70% lower prevalence of Alzheimer's disease than a control group.

Is there an association between 'normal' glucose levels and coronary heart disease?

Although diabetes is a strong risk factor for coronary heart disease, the association between glycaemia in the 'normal' range and coronary heart disease has previously been controversial. However, a recent study shows that glycosylated haemoglobin levels are positively correlated with the risk of future coronary heart disease independent of BMI, cholesterol, age, sex, blood pressure or smoking history *(BMJ 2001;322:15–18)*.

This study looked at 4,662 men aged between 45 and 79 years old and found that HbA_{1C} concentration significantly predicted all-cause mortality, even below the threshold commonly accepted for diagnosis of diabetes. This implies that glucose control for coronary heart disease should begin in patients with impaired glucose tolerance. Yet, there is still no trial to confirm that improved glycaemic control will reduce the risk of coronary heart disease in people without diabetes. It is possible that glucose is merely a marker for other risk factors rather than a causal risk factor for cardiovascular disease.

Should patients receive ramipril?
It is well established that treating hypertension reduces the risk of CHD. In a recent trial, the HOPE study, patients at high risk of cardiovascular events were given the ACE inhibitor ramipril *(NEMJ 2000;342;145–53)*. This resulted in a 22% reduction in the combined end point of cardiovascular death, non-fatal myocardial infarction and stroke. These benefits were similar in normotensive and hypertensive patients. From this it could therefore be argued that all patients at a high risk of CHD should receive ramipril!

Is there any evidence to support cardiac rehabilitation?
Meta-analyses of randomised trials have shown that cardiac rehabilitation after myocardial infarction reduces mortality by 20–24%. Clinical guidelines for cardiac rehabilitation have been published by the Royal College of Physicians but currently less than half of patients receive any form of rehabilitation. Disadvantaged social groups include women, the elderly and ethnic minorities.

Is exercise beneficial?
Regular exercise has numerous benefits, including reducing hypertension and CHD. Short bouts of exercise can be just as effective at protecting the heart as longer workouts, but getting the heart rate up is a key factor because light activity offers no cardiac benefit, as two new studies have shown *(Circulation 2000;102:975-80, 981–7)*.

One of the biggest barriers for implementing evidence-based practice may be convincing patients that they need to take part in life-long prevention from coronary heart disease. In one study, 30% of patients declined to participate in a nurse-led prevention programme *(BMJ 1998;316:1434-7)*. Patients often perceive a 'heart attack' to be an acute, self-limiting condition rather than the onset of a high-risk chronic disease.

In summary, therefore, it is important that GP teams are able to identify

Chronic Diseases

all people with established CHD and all people who are at significant risk of CHD but who have not yet developed symptoms. Both groups should then be offered the appropriate advice and treatment to reduce their risks in the future. It is very likely that secondary-prevention clinics will be organised at a primary care group level, which will facilitate the delivery of various aspects of the national service framework for coronary heart disease and improve standards of care across the country.

 USEFUL WEBSITES

www.bcs.com – British Cardiac Society
www.pccs.org.uk – Primary Care Cardiovascular Society
www.hyp.ac.uk/bhs – British Hypertension Society (Includes copies of CVD risk charts)
www.cardiacrehabilitation.org.uk – information regarding rehabilitation

ACRONYMS OF IMPORTANT CARDIOVASCULAR TRIALS

MONICA	-	Monitoring trends and determinants in cardiovascular disease
4S	-	Scandinavian Simvastatin Survival Study
CARE	-	Cholesterol and Recurrent Events trial
LIPID	-	The Long-term Intervention with Pravastatin in Ischaemic Disease
WOSCOPS	-	West of Scotland Coronary Prevention Study
HOPE	-	The Heart Outcomes Prevention Evaluation

SUMMARY POINTS OF CORONARY HEART DISEASE

Always consider:
- Smoking status
- Weight
- Exercise
- Blood pressure
- Aspirin
- Statins

Chronic Diseases

THE CORONARY HEART DISEASE NATIONAL SERVICE FRAMEWORK

This was published by the Department of Health in March 2000 and has been designed to 'transform the prevention, diagnosis and treatment of coronary heart disease'.

Coronary heart disease is one of the most common causes of death in the UK. More than 1.4 million people suffer from angina, and 300,000 people have heart attacks every year. Heart disease is much more common in deprived areas, yet treatment and care are often better in more prosperous areas. This 'postcode' lottery of care is unacceptable and the NSF attempts to end it.

What do National Service Frameworks (NSFs) do?
National Service Frameworks have been created to set national standards and define service models for a specific service or care group, put in place programmes to support implementation and establish performance measures against which progress within an agreed timescale will be measured. This is the second NSF to be produced.

What does the CHD NSF state?
This framework sets out a programme designed to achieve the government target of cutting coronary heart disease and stroke by an ambitious 40% by 2010. It sets 12 standards for the prevention, diagnosis and treatment of coronary heart disease; describes service models; and explains how the standards can be delivered and how progress will be monitored, with milestones and goals.

The funding implications are enormous. The Government has provided a £50m package to kick start the programme, which will mainly be used for defibrillators, chest pain clinics and ambulances.

These 12 standards include:
- Setting up 50 rapid access chest pain clinics, patients to be seen within two weeks of referral
- Reduction in the 'call to needle' time for thrombolysis (75% of patients within 30 minutes by April 2002)
- Improved ambulance response times (75% of emergency calls will have to receive a response, with defibrillators, within 8 minutes)
- Improved use of effective medicines (90% of patients post MI

Chronic Diseases

should be discharged on statins, aspirin and beta blockers)
- Increase in the total annual number of revascularisation procedures (to provide an extra 3,000 nationally)
- Introduction of specialist smoking cessation clinics by Health Authorities
- Development of policies to reduce incidence of CHD in the community

What does this mean for GPs?
From April 2001 all practices should have a register of CHD patients and provide structured care with nationally accepted guidelines. GP teams also have to identify patients who are at risk of coronary heart disease and offer them appropriate advice and treatment to reduce their risks. Regular audits on this information have to be performed. This is obviously going to involve a considerable amount of work in many practices but is important, as these measures are a start towards improving the quality of care for patients with ischaemic heart disease.

What are the negative parts of this NSF?
This is a very lengthy document consisting of 124 pages, with another 283 pages containing eight appendices! It is written with a lot of repetition and contains a large amount of 'management jargon' which is not always easy to follow. The main document is not referenced although it does claim to provide evidence-based advice. However, it may be worth noting that there is no current available evidence to support the establishment of chest pain clinics.

Many of the current deficiencies in providing adequate secondary prevention care in coronary heart disease patients is often due to poor funding; for example, low prescription rates for statins, long waiting times for exercise ECGs and angiograms. It is unclear how holding regular audits will actually improve this! The NSF has been described as a blueprint for audit rather than a guideline for patient management and the main audit burden is going to fall on General Practices.

 USEFUL WEBSITE

www.doh.gov.uk/nsf/coronary.htm

Chronic Diseases

📋 SUMMARY POINTS FOR THE CHD NSF

- ❖ 12 standards covered in NSF
- ❖ Aim to reduce heart disease
- ❖ Involve primary and secondary care
- ❖ Clear and challenging targets

AIMS OF THE NATIONAL SERVICE FRAMEWORK

- ❖ Create disease registers
- ❖ Produce locally agreed protocols
- ❖ Provide structured care
- ❖ Perform regular audits

Chronic Diseases

HEART FAILURE

Heart failure, like hypertension, is a very common but poorly managed condition. 50% of patients with heart failure are undetected, 50% of those detected are not treated and 50% of those treated are not adequately controlled.

Despite improvements in treatment the prognosis for patients with heart failure remains poor; the risk of death annually is 5–10% in patients with mild symptoms and 30–40% in those with advanced disease.

There is a poor correlation between symptoms and signs of heart failure and echocardiogram findings. In addition, although the echocardiogram is the gold standard investigation for heart failure, GPs are limited by its availability. Lack of resources (e.g. echocardiography) and expertise are the great barriers to efficient treatment of heart failure.

What are the best treatments for heart failure?

There are now so many different drugs known to benefit patients with heart failure that treatment can often become confusing and complex for both the patient and the doctor.

Diuretics

For many years, diuretics have been an important part of symptomatic treatment for patients with heart failure and evidence of fluid retention. However, their long-term effects on mortality rates and other endpoints are not known (it would now be unethical to trial).

Angiotensin converting enzyme (ACE) inhibitors

ACE inhibitors have been evaluated extensively in randomised controlled trials (e.g. CONSENSUS, RESOLVD studies) in a large number of patients with heart failure and were found to reduce mortality and morbidity. Benefits also extend to different patient groups, such as elderly patients, women, patients with or without coronary artery disease, with different degrees of functional impairment and with a history of use of diuretics and digoxin. In the absence of clear contraindications these drugs should therefore be used as first-line agents in all patients with left ventricular dysfunction who have or do not have symptoms.

However, less than half of patients with heart failure in the community are receiving ACE inhibitors and patients taking them often do not have their renal function measured *(BMJ 1999;318:234–7)*. It has been recommended that patients should be screened for risk factors predisposing them to uraemia (for example old age, peripheral vascular disease or concomitant treatment with non-steroidal drugs). Renal function should be checked before and 7–10 days after ACE inhibitors are started in all patients and thereafter annually only in those with risk factors. It has also been proposed that fear of side-effects may be a major barrier to ACE inhibitor use by General Practitioners; however the introduction of these drugs has been shown to cause problems very rarely *(BMJ 2000;321:1113–6)*.

Angiotensin II receptor antagonists
The ELITE II study *(J Card Fail 1999;5:146–54)* confirmed the benefit of these drugs. They are mainly used in patients who are intolerant of ACE inhibitors, usually because of a cough.

Beta-blockers
Beta-blockers have been evaluated in nearly 10,000 patients with chronic heart failure in over 20 randomised clinical trials (e.g. MERIT-HF and CIBIS-II trials) and have been shown to decrease the risk of death and the need for hospital admission. These benefits were attained in patients already taking ACE inhibitors and diuretics, with ischaemic and non-ischaemic disease and with different degrees of functional impairment, although clinical trials have generally carefully selected stable patients.

Even in carefully selected and treated patients there is often an initial deterioration in symptoms, followed frequently by subsequent improvement. Owing to the complexities of initiating, titrating and monitoring treatment with beta-blockers in heart failure, this treatment should generally be given only by experienced doctors or in specialised clinics. The choice of beta-blocker (selective versus non-selective versus carvedilol) remains controversial and is currently under investigation in randomised trials.

Digoxin
There is some evidence that digoxin can provide some symptomatic benefit in patients in sinus rhythm with heart failure. However, it does not appear to improve mortality *(NEMJ 1997;336:525–33)*.

Spironolactone
The RALES study *(Lancet 1999;341:709–17)* showed that patients who

Chronic Diseases

received spironolactone in addition to their usual treatment had a decreased mortality of 30%. The patients in this study had severe heart failure persisting despite standard therapy. More trials are needed before spironolactone can be recommended as a routine treatment for heart failure.

General Practitioners have a vital role in the early detection and treatment of the main risk factors for heart failure, namely hypertension and ischaemic heart disease, and other cardiovascular risk factors, such as smoking and hyperlipidaemia. The Framingham study has shown a decline in hypertension as a risk factor for heart failure over the years, which probably reflects improvements in treatment. Early detection of left ventricular dysfunction in 'high risk' asymptomatic patients, for example those who have hypertension or atrial fibrillation, and treatment with angiotensin converting enzyme inhibitors can minimise the progression to symptomatic heart failure.

ACRONYMS OF IMPORTANT CARDIOVASCULAR TRIALS

CONSENSUS	-	Co-operative North Scandinavian Enalapril Survival Study
RESOLVD	-	Randomised Evaluation of Strategies for Left Ventricular Dysfunction
ELITE	-	Evaluation of Losartan in the Elderly study
MERIF-HF	-	Metoprolol CR/XL Randomised Intervention Trial in Congestive Heart Failure
CIBIS	-	The Cardiac Insufficiency Bisoprolol Study
RALES	-	Randomized Aldactone Evaluation Study

SUMMARY POINTS FOR HEART FAILURE

- ❖ Heart failure is underdetected and undertreated
- ❖ Affects 10% of people over 75 years old
- ❖ ACE inhibitors are standard treatment
- ❖ Target risk factors in all patients

ATRIAL FIBRILLATION

There is an increased incidence of atrial fibrillation with increasing age, one study suggests a prevalence of 2.4% in patients over the age of 50 years *(BJGP 1997;47:285–9)*. Atrial fibrillation is an independent risk factor for developing a stroke; its presence increases the risk of stroke five-fold. Patients with atrial fibrillation who do sustain a stroke have a higher mortality rate, greater disability, a longer duration of hospital stay and a lower rate of discharge to their own home. Community based studies, however, show that atrial fibrillation is still underdiagnosed and undertreated.

Should patients with atrial fibrillation be prescribed warfarin?

It is recommended that patients who are at a high risk of stroke should be identified and targeted for anticoagulation in the absence of contraindications *(Lancet 1999;353:4–6)*, see Table on page 18. This risk should be reviewed at regular intervals, at least annually. High-risk patients should receive warfarin (INR 2.0–3.0) if possible, patients at moderate risk should receive either warfarin or aspirin, depending on each individual case and low-risk patients should receive aspirin.

Randomised trials have established that anticoagulation with warfarin is associated with a relative reduction in risk of stroke of 68% *(Lancet 1996;648:633–8)*. Aspirin has been shown to be less effective in stroke reduction among high-risk patients, but is more convenient and theoretically safer then warfarin. A recent systematic review of long-term anticoagulation and aspirin in patients with AF showed for the first time that aspirin is probably as effective at preventing fatal and non-fatal cardiovascular events as warfarin *(BMJ 2001;322:321–4)*. However, larger trials need to be undertaken before a change in the current practice can be recommended. There is no evidence that adding aspirin to warfarin confers any additional benefit.

Although anticoagulation in those aged over 75 is associated with greater risk when the international normalised ratio (INR) is maintained at 2.0–4.5, the SPAF III (Stroke Prevention in Atrial Fibrillation) trial showed that anticoagulation to a lower INR of 1.5–3.0 is both safe and effective in reducing the risk of stroke in this age group.

Why are some patients with atrial fibrillation not anticoagulated?

Despite evidence in published literature, anticoagulation is underused in clinical practice, partly because it was not known whether trial efficacy

Chronic Diseases

translates into clinical practice. The patients in the trials were highly selected and had very close monitoring and follow-up. The trials were designed to provide an estimate of treatment efficacy but have been widely interpreted as being studies of warfarin treatment. There is a counter-argument that the benefits of warfarin were actually underestimated, since patients randomised to the warfarin arms of the studies who actually did sustain a stroke often had subtherapeutic INRs.

However, a recent community based study showed that stroke and haemorrhage rates were comparable to those in randomised studies *(BMJ 2000;320:1236–39)*.

Other reasons for the poor prescribing of warfarin in atrial fibrillation patients may include concern over cerebral haemorrhage, the problems associated with initiating therapy in elderly housebound patients and the inconvenience of safely monitoring anticoagulation in the community. A recent small study demonstrated that patients on warfarin could manage their INR at home as safely as at a hospital anticoagulation clinic *(Lancet 2000;356:97–102)*. This was made possible by reliable, easy-to-use machines using capillary blood samples. Longer-term studies are needed to assess the feasibility of this but home management would obviously have many advantages.

A recent study of elderly patients in General Practice showed that nearly 40% of patients with atrial fibrillation preferred not to receive anticoagulation when they were given information about stroke risk and consequences *(BMJ 2000;320:1380–84)*. The findings of this study suggest that guidelines for the management of atrial fibrillation should be modified to incorporate patients' preferences in treatment decisions, particularly with regard to the consequences of anticoagulation treatment.

Chronic Diseases

RISK OF STROKE IN NON-RHEUMATIC ATRIAL FIBRILLATION

High Risk (12% annually)
All patients with previous history of TIA or CVA
All patients aged over 75 years with diabetes, hypertension or ischaemic heart disease
All patients with clinical evidence of valve disease or heart failure

Medium Risk (8% annually)
All patients under 65 years with diabetes, hypertension or ischaemic heart disease
All patients over 65 years who have not been identified in the high risk group

Low Risk (1% annually)
All other patients under 65 years

SUMMARY POINTS FOR ATRIAL FIBRILLATION

❖ Risk of AF increases with age
❖ Associated with five-fold risk of stroke
❖ Patients at high risk of stroke need warfarin

Chronic Diseases

STROKE

Stroke is the third highest cause of death in the UK and the biggest single cause of major disability. Treatment in the UK is far from satisfactory. Stroke can occur at any age, but half of all strokes occur in people aged over 70 years. About 80% of all acute strokes are caused by cerebral infarction; the remainder are caused by haemorrhage. More than 50% of patients are physically dependent on others six months after a stroke.

Health care providers in the UK are beginning to address the poor services for stroke patients. In April 2000, the Royal College of Physicians produced a national strategy for stroke in an attempt to improve stroke services in England, Wales and Northern Ireland, which have been criticised as disorganised, haphazard and poor. The Department of Health has developed a National Service Framework for elderly people, which focuses on stroke.

The national clinical guidelines for stroke are the first comprehensive guidelines to cover all aspects of stroke care from diagnosis to rehabilitation. They also include the views of patients and carers on what they want from stroke services.

The European Stroke Initiative (EUSI) has also recently published its recommendations for management of stroke *(Cerebrovasc Dis 2000;10:335–51)* which are largely similar to the Royal College of Physician guidelines.

Recommendations

All patients should be seen by specialised teams
There is strong evidence that patients treated in stroke units are less likely to die and more likely to recover fully or partially from a stroke *(BMJ 1997;314:1151–9)*. Multidisciplinary teams should co-ordinate stroke care in the community. Currently less than a quarter of patients are being treated in specialist stroke units.

Interventions for acute ischaemic stroke
These are summarised in the box on page 21. Early use of aspirin (300 mg) reduces the chance of death and dependency and improves the chance of complete recovery *(Lancet 1997;349:1569–81)*. There has been no evidence to show that immediate anticoagulation is beneficial.

19

Chronic Diseases

Thrombolysis trials have shown very conflicting results. Tissue plasminogen activator (tPA) can reduce the risk of dependency but it increases the risk of death (from intracerebral haemorrhage and from any cause). It is recommended that tPA is only given in specialist centres, within three hours of the stroke and as part of randomised controlled trials.

Carers and their families
They must be involved in decision making and have their own individual and psychological needs regularly reviewed.

Secondary prevention
The main interventions with proven benefit are aspirin, cholesterol reduction in patients with existing coronary heart disease and carotid endarterectomy in people with severe carotid artery stenosis. In addition, people with atrial fibrillation have been shown to benefit from oral anticoagulation (or aspirin in the case of contraindications to anticoagulants).

Hypertension persisting after one month should be treated according to the British Hypertension Society guidelines. All patients should receive aspirin (if there are contraindications then dipyridamole or clopidogrel could be considered). The effect of reducing cholesterol in patients with a prior stroke but no history of coronary heart disease is, as yet, still uncertain.

Primary prevention
Hypertension is the most prevalent and modifiable risk factor for stroke in primary prevention, with its treatment substantially reducing the risk of stroke. The risk factors for stroke are similar to those for coronary heart disease so primary care teams have a very important role in primary stroke prevention.

Many trials continue to be conducted in this very important area of clinical practice and it is likely that options for stroke treatment will continue to expand in the future.

National Service Framework for Elderly People and Stroke
Stroke is covered in Standard Five of the NSF, which was published in March 2001. This aims to reduce the incidence of stroke in the population and ensure that those who have had a stroke have prompt access to integrated stroke care services. It states there are four components for the development of integrated stroke services:

Chronic Diseases

1. Prevention: Including identification, treatment and follow-up of those at risk of stroke.
2. Immediate care: Including care from a specialist stroke team.
3. Early and continuing rehabilitation.
4. Long-term support for the stroke patient and their carers.

By 2004 Primary Care Trusts will have to use protocols to identify, treat and refer stroke patients and every General Practice will have established clinical audit systems for stroke. In addition, by April 2002 all hospitals are to have plans to introduce a specialist stroke service. It is still unclear at present how this is going to be fully implemented. Success can obviously only be achieved if there is adequate provision of staff, education, training and finance to carry out the programme.

INTERVENTIONS FOR ACUTE ISCHAEMIC STROKE

Beneficial
Stroke units
Aspirin

Trade-off between benefits and harms
Thrombolytic treatment

Likely to be ineffective or harmful
Immediate systemic anticoagulation
Acute reduction of blood pressure

 USEFUL WEBSITES

www.rcplondon.ac.uk/college/ceeu_stroke_home.htm – Stroke guidelines
www.dcn.ed.ac.uk/csrg – Cochrane Stroke group website
www.nottingham.ac.uk/stroke-medicine – British Association of Stroke Physicians
www.doh.gov.uk/nsf/olderpeople.htm – National Service Framework for Older People

Chronic Diseases

DIABETES MELLITUS

The prevalence of diagnosed diabetes within the UK is about 3%. Diabetes is a very common disease and its incidence is rising, especially as a result of the expanding ageing population (more than 10% of people over 65 years are diabetic) and an increasing incidence of obesity. Diabetes is 3–4 times more common amongst people of Asian, African and African-Caribbean descent – up to 25% of people of Asian origin aged over 60 have diabetes.

Diabetes is a leading cause of blindness, kidney failure and limb amputation and greatly increases the risk of coronary heart disease and stroke. Diabetes accounts for at least 8% of acute sector costs – it has been estimated that the average cost of in-patient care for a person with diabetes is more than six times that for a person who does not have diabetes.

How is the diagnosis of diabetes confirmed?
The World Health Organisation introduced new criteria for the definition, diagnosis and classification of diabetes in June 2000. They recommend that the cut-off point for diagnosing diabetes using a fasting plasma glucose level should be lowered from 7.8 to **7.0 mmol/l**. The new criteria set out methods for diagnosing diabetes.

The methods for diagnosing diabetes are as follows:

With symptoms (polyuria, thirst, unexplained weight loss)
*   A random venous plasma glucose concentration ≥ 11.1 mmol/l **or**
*   A fasting venous plasma glucose concentration ≥ 7.0 mmol/l **or**
*   2 hour venous plasma glucose concentration ≥ 11.1 mmol/l
    2 hours after 75 g anhydrous glucose in an oral glucose tolerance test (OGTT)

With no symptoms
*   Diagnosis must **not** be based on a single glucose determination. At least one additional glucose result on another day with a value in the diabetic range is essential. This can be either fasting, from a random sample or from the 2 hour OGTT. If the fasting or random values are not diagnostic, the 2 hour value should be used.

There is some concern about the implications of these changes for diabetes care; earlier diagnosis will increase the total number of people

Chronic Diseases

with diabetes but most of these will be diet controlled. In the long term, complications should be reduced to the benefit of the individual and to the health service.

Why is diabetes important in primary care?

GPs have a pivotal role to play in ensuring that people with diabetes receive effective diabetes care. It is usually the GP who makes the initial diagnosis of diabetes and it is the GP who, in consultation with other members of the specialist diabetes team, is responsible for agreeing with patients where they receive each element of care.

Diabetes care has been shown to be as good in primary care as that provided in secondary care, especially in practices where a GP has a special interest in diabetes and the care provided is well organised and integrated. 75% of diabetic patients are currently routinely managed in primary care.

A report by the Audit Commission recently revealed that there is a wide variation in the standard of diabetes care across the country. It found that secondary care diabetes services are stretched, with waiting times for first appointments up to 14 weeks, and many patient complaints of long clinic waits and insufficient time with clinical staff. It is therefore very unlikely that secondary care will be able to cope with the expanding numbers of diabetic patients.

A recent national survey of diabetes care in General Practices showed that the majority of practices require further training and education about diabetes *(BJGP 2000;50:542–5)*. The National Service Framework for diabetes is going to be produced in 2001, which should hopefully improve the standards of care. It is likely to suggest that primary care takes on the routine care of most patients with diabetes. More resources and financial incentives will be needed for this to be delivered.

A revised edition of Diabetes UK's *'Recommendations for the Management of Diabetes in Primary Care'* was published in October 2000 and is intended to assist all those professionals involved in the care of people with diabetes. The emphasis in this document is primarily on the organisation of care, rather than on the clinical management of diabetes and is available on the Diabetes UK website (see page 27).

Chronic Diseases

What are the key elements of effective diabetes care?
These can be summarised as having
- A planned programme of care for all patients with diabetes
- Clear management plans agreed with each patient, tailored to meet the needs of the individual and their carers
- Practice-based diabetes registers to facilitate regular call and recall of patients

Healthcare professionals have a responsibility to provide appropriate education to equip people with diabetes with the knowledge, skills, attitudes and motivation to manage their diabetes care effectively and to modify their lifestyle in such a way as to maximise their well-being.

Is there evidence that improved glycaemic control leads to a reduction in complications?
There is increasing evidence to confirm that meticulous glycaemic control can prevent or delay the onset of the complications of diabetes. The impact of these complications can also be greatly reduced if they are detected early and appropriately managed. Thus, regular surveillance for diabetes and early diagnosis of the complications of diabetes are also important.

There are two very important studies regarding this.

DCCT (Diabetes Control & Complications Trial)
This is an important study, which demonstrated that patients receiving intensive insulin treatment for their diabetes had fewer microvascular complications *(Diabetes 1996;45:1289–98)*. Long-term follow up of these patients was later published *(NEMJ 2000;342:381–5)* which showed that these benefits persist. However, the improved glycaemic control was not completely advantageous to patients as it resulted in the need for more frequent BM testing and increased frequency of insulin injections. Many patients also gained weight and had an increased frequency of hypoglycaemic episodes so it actually resulted in a huge disruption to their lifestyles.

UKPDS (UK Prospective Diabetes Study)
This was a massive study involving over 5,000 Type 2 diabetic patients over a 20 year period, which studied whether intensive control of blood glucose after diagnosis of diabetes was beneficial *(Lancet 1998; 353:837–53)*. It demonstrated that better glycaemic control reduced microvascular complications and intense management of cardiovascular

Chronic Diseases

risk factors reduced macrovascular complications. Essentially, the lower the levels of blood glucose, HbA_{1C} and BP; the lower the risk of complications.

Should there be a screening programme for Type 2 diabetes?
The UKPDS study also showed that about 50% of patients had early signs of complications at the time of diagnosis of their diabetes. This therefore raises the question as to whether screening for diabetes should be introduced, i.e. if diabetes is diagnosed earlier then theoretically there would be a reduced incidence of complications. This issue is clearly discussed in a recent BMJ Education and Debate article *(BMJ 2001;322:986–8)*. This article concludes that at present, there is no justification for universal screening for diabetes in the UK. However, there is some support for screening and intensive treatment in population subgroups in whom undiagnosed diabetes is especially prevalent and cardiovascular risk is high, provided the systems for organisation and management are optimised.

Primary care teams will play an important part in helping those with diabetes achieve better control and detect the earliest signs of complications, through regular systematic surveillance.

How important is treating hypertension in diabetic patients?
A recent study using the UKPDS data showed that **any** reduction in blood pressure for Type 2 diabetic patients reduces the risk of complications *(BMJ 2000;321:412–20)*. Intensive BP control is at least as (probably even more) important than intensive treatment of glucose levels in the reduction of complications in diabetic patients. The blood pressure target from the UKPDS study has been set at 140/80.

It has been estimated that the number of diabetics taking anti-hypertensive medication would need to **double** in order to meet the targets of 140/80!

Results from the HOPE (Heart Outcomes Prevention Evaluation) study also showed that adding ramipril to the drug regimen of high-risk diabetic patients provides vascular-protective and reno-protective effects independent of its effect on hypertension *(Lancet 2000;355:253–9)*.

Do diabetic patients have a higher risk of cardiovascular disease?
Patients with diabetes, especially Type 2, have a greatly increased risk of cardiovascular disease compared with non-diabetics. This is clearly

Chronic Diseases

illustrated in the Joint British Societies Coronary Risk Prediction charts. Four out of five deaths in patients with Type 2 diabetes are caused by cardiovascular disease. It is important to institute statin therapy and aspirin in patients with Type 2 diabetes and established cardiovascular disease. The current recommendation is to prescribe statins to patients with a 30% risk over 10 years of a CHD event.

In view of the high risk of cardiovascular disease in people with diabetes, particularly those with Type 2 diabetes, the careful management of other cardiovascular risk factors, including smoking, physical inactivity, obesity and especially hypertension, in their annual diabetes review is essential.

What new drugs are available for diabetic patients?
A new class of drugs for Type 2 diabetics called glitazones have recently been introduced; rosiglitazone (Avandia) and pioglitazone (Actos) were launched in 2000. They work by reducing the body's resistance to the action of insulin and enable a more efficient use of insulin. They are licensed for combination use with a sulphonylurea or metformin (they are contraindicated for use with insulin).

These new agents offer a real alternative in the treatment of obese patients who do not achieve sufficient blood glucose control with metformin. They are expected to postpone the need for insulin therapy in Type 2 diabetics for some years. They also hold out the possibility that through treatment of insulin resistance, the macrovascular complications of Type 2 diabetes may be reduced.

What does all this mean for patients?
It is well known that in practice it is very difficult to maintain any reductions in glucose concentrations and blood pressure, even when multiple drugs are used in combination. It is a daunting prospect for any diabetic patient to consider taking metformin, ramipril, simvastatin, aspirin, other oral hypoglycaemics and other antihypertensives on a regular basis! The compliance of diabetic patients is poorer than expected – a recent study presented at the British Diabetic Association Annual Conference collected anonymous information on prescriptions from diabetic patients in Dundee and it showed that only 1 in 3 of patients comply with single medications and about 1 in 10 comply with two medications!

The future of diabetes care in the UK will be challenging to primary care. Although clear therapeutic goals have been defined, doctors may need to negotiate realistic goals with individual patients regarding their optimal treatment.

 USEFUL WEBSITES

www.diabetes.org.uk – Diabetes UK (formally the British Diabetic Association)
www.audit-commission.gov.uk – Audit Commission report
www.nsc.nhs.uk – National Screening Committee website – evaluation of Type 2 diabetes mellitus screening against the National Screening Committee Handbook criteria

---

SUMMARY POINTS FOR DIABETES

- Incidence of diabetes is rising
- New criteria for diagnosis of diabetes (June 2000)
- 75% diabetic patients are routinely managed in primary care
- Meticulous glycaemic control can reduce complications
- Careful management of other cardiovascular risk factors is essential
- NSF for diabetes is still awaited

Chronic Diseases

OSTEOPOROSIS

Osteoporosis is defined as a skeletal disease characterised by low bone mass and deterioration of the microarchitecture of bone tissue, which makes bone more fragile and increases the risk of fracture.

Osteoporosis affects approximately 40% of women over 70 years of age in the UK. It is emerging as one of the biggest health problems in postmenopausal women – resulting in more deaths in older women than cancer of the cervix, uterus and ovaries combined. The annual cost to the NHS of osteoporotic fractures has been estimated at £940m. Approximately 20% of patients die within a year of sustaining a fractured neck of the femur as a result of osteoporosis.

A low level of awareness of the benefits of early identification for risk factors, together with the pressure to reduce prescribing costs, often results in ineffective disease management. It is not surprising therefore that any clinical interventions to both prevent and treat osteoporosis have been very topical recently.

How are patients at high risk of osteoporosis identified?

Osteoporosis can be reliably identified by bone densitometry, which is still the gold standard for both the measurement of disease and the response to therapy. Unfortunately, the availability of dual energy X–ray absorptiometry (DEXA) scanning machines is still very variable across the UK, despite only costing the NHS £20–45 per scan. DEXA scans have been shown to predict future fracture rate with a high specificity and low sensitivity. It is recommended that DEXA scanning should be used for patients at a high risk of developing osteoporosis rather than for screening of the general population (see box on page 31).

A previous fragility fracture is a strong independent risk for further fracture and is, in itself, an indication for treatment for osteoporosis without the need for bone mineral density measurement. However, a recent audit found that most patients who have an osteoporotic fracture are not started on treatment for secondary prevention of osteoporosis *(Ann Rheum Dis 1998; 57:378–9)*.

How important is corticosteroid-induced osteoporosis?

In most patients taking an oral corticosteroid long term, there is a fall in bone mass and bone mineral density. Longitudinal studies have shown that the most rapid rate of bone loss occurs in the first year of treatment

Chronic Diseases

and thereafter bone loss continues at a rate of two to three times normal on long-term therapy in older subjects. As many as 40% of patients on long-term steroids may develop a fracture secondary to osteoporosis.

The exact dose of corticosteroid that induces clinically significant bone loss is not yet well established. Studies in patients have consistently demonstrated a clinically important fall in bone density in patients taking 7.5 mg prednisolone a day. One study indicated that only 14% of patients treated with oral corticosteroids are also prescribed therapy to prevent bone loss *(BMJ 1996; 313:344–6)*.

The National Osteoporosis Society has produced guidelines on the management of glucocorticoid-induced osteoporosis, which, where possible, are based on current clinical evidence (see website details page 31). In the UK, the most commonly used therapies for glucocorticoid-induced osteoporosis are hormone replacement therapy and bisphosphonates.

What drug interventions can be used to prevent and treat osteoporosis?
The Royal College of Physicians issued guidelines in 1999 for the prevention and treatment of osteoporosis. In the 18 months following the release of these guidelines, new clinical trial data became available for existing and new pharmacological interventions and so an 'Update on pharmacological interventions for the prevention and treatment of osteoporosis' has been prepared by the original Guidelines Writing Group, in collaboration with the Bone and Tooth Society, and endorsed by the Royal College of Physicians. This report also includes a useful algorithm for the management of individual patients, derived from an evidence-based synthesis of different pharmacological interventions.

Prophylaxis against osteoporosis obviously needs to be continued long-term. There is no evidence that bone protection lasts much beyond current use for any treatment option, so long-term costs (both to the patient and financially) have to be considered. The side-effects and method of administration must therefore be acceptable to the patient if compliance is to be optimal. Thus the increasing range of treatments and the greater acceptability of these options are very important.

Bisphosphonates
Cyclical etidronate (Didronel), alendronate (Fosamax) and risedronate (Actonel) are all licensed for the prevention and treatment of osteoporosis (and corticosteroid-induced osteoporosis). There are, at

Chronic Diseases

present, no randomised controlled trials comparing the relative efficacy of these agents. Generally, cyclical etidronate may be best for patients with mainly lumbar spine disease and alendronate is beneficial in patients with more severe disease, involving both lumbar spine and femoral neck (and also for patients who may prefer once-weekly therapy). The optimal duration of treatment with bisphosphonates has not yet been established.

Selective oestrogen receptor modulator therapy (SERMs)
Raloxifene mimics the beneficial effects of oestrogen on the bone but blocks the oestrogen effect on the uterus and breast tissue. The effect in reducing vertebral fractures with raloxifene is similar to that of bisphosphonates and the effect on BMD is similar to that of oestrogens. It does not cause uterine bleeding or gastrointestinal side-effects, and does not raise concerns about breast disease (*JAMA 1999;282:637–45*). The precise place for raloxifene in the prevention and management of osteoporosis in General Practice is still a matter for debate.

Hormone replacement therapy (HRT)
Earlier assumptions that taking HRT would reduce the risk of fracture in the future have unfortunately not been confirmed; oestrogen-induced skeletal benefits probably disappear within 6–10 years of stopping treatment. Therefore, women would need to take oestrogens from their menopause until at least their early seventies to reduce their risk of osteoporotic fractures.

Oestrogen can be a cost-effective treatment option for postmenopausal women. However, there are no data on vertebral fracture reduction rates and oestrogen may be an unattractive option for many elderly women. In addition, the efficacy of HRT is mainly from observational studies, which are likely to overestimate the beneficial effects.

Calcium and Vitamin D
Calcium and vitamin D supplements may slow down the rate of bone loss in elderly women who already have a low BMD. However, in patients with established osteoporosis this effect is not enough. However, calcium can complement the other treatments (SERMs, bisphosphonates, oestrogen). It is recommended that those people at risk of osteoporosis should maintain an adequate intake of calcium and vitamin D, and any deficiency should be corrected by increasing dietary intake or taking supplements. Elderly patients, especially those in residential or nursing homes, may routinely benefit from supplements.

Chronic Diseases

Statins
Finally, a recent observation found that inhibition of hydroxymethylglutaryl coenzyme A reductase with statin therapy may reduce the risk of fracture *(JAMA 2000;283:3205–10)*. This therefore raises the possibility that patients requiring statins for their cardiovascular disease may derive additional benefit in terms of osteoporosis prevention!

RISK FACTORS FOR OSTEOPOROSIS

- Early menopause
- Hysterectomy < 45 years
- Long-term prednisolone ≥ 7.5mg/day
- Malabsorption disorder (e.g. coeliac disease)
- Premenopausal episodes of amenorrhoea
- Lean body habitus
- Strong family history
- Cigarette smoking

 USEFUL WEBSITES

www.rcplondon.ac.uk – Royal College of Physicians
www.nos.org.uk – National Osteoporosis Society

SUMMARY POINTS FOR OSTEOPOROSIS

- Annual cost of osteoporosis to NHS is £940 million
- Often underdiagnosed and suboptimally managed
- Several effective medical interventions available
- Poor compliance with treatment is a problem

CHAPTER 2: RESPIRATORY DISEASES

ASTHMA

Asthma is still underdiagnosed and poorly treated despite an increased awareness of the condition. Most patients with asthma are managed in primary care. The British Thoracic Society Guidelines are an example of very successful guidelines and are due to be updated soon.

What is changing about inhalers?

All CFC inhalers are to be replaced by CFC-free inhalers. This transition has been slower than originally predicted as there has been a lack of appropriate alternatives. CFC-free inhalers are different shapes so will not fit into patients' spacers which adds to the confusion. Steroid inhalers are difficult to reformulate; the beclomethasone formulation currently licensed in the UK (beclomethasone dipropionate) has increased lung deposition and is licensed at half the standard beclomethasone dose.

How safe are inhaled steroids?

The amount of inhaled steroid absorbed in the body is very low but systemic side-effects can occur – e.g. osteoporosis, growth retardation and cataracts. Side-effects are unlikely with low-dose inhaled steroids (< 400 mcg/day beclomethasone in children and < 1000 mcg/day in adults). All children receiving inhaled steroids should have their height measured regularly and any children needing high maintenance doses are best supervised by a paediatrician. Children with viral associated wheeze should not be prescribed inhaled steroids. The most important safeguard for patients is to have their asthma controlled regularly and the dose of inhaled steroid is stepped down once control of symptoms is achieved *(DTB Jan 2000)*.

What are the NICE guidelines for childhood asthma?

In August 2000, NICE produced guidelines for the use of inhaler devices in children under 5 years with chronic asthma. The main recommendations are:
- Pressurised metered dose inhalers with a spacer system (with a facemask if necessary)
- In children aged 3 to 5 years a dry powder could be considered
- Choice on inhaler should be governed by specific individual need and likelihood of good compliance

Which new drugs are available to treat asthma?

Leukotriene receptor antagonists montelukast (Singulair) and zafirlukast

Respiratory Diseases

(Accolate) are a new class of oral asthma therapies that have anti-inflammatory and bronchodilator properties. They have been introduced since the National Asthma Guidelines were written in 1995. Currently they seem to be best used as add-ons to low or high-dose inhaled steroids where control of persistent asthma symptoms has not been achieved (Steps 3 and 4 of the guidelines).

Do self-management plans have a role in asthma management?
Asthma lends itself to the use of guided self-management plans based on the BTS guidelines. There is plenty of evidence which shows that the use of self-management plans for asthma can lead to a reduction in hospitalisation rates, time off work and improvement in symptom control. Nurses with advanced qualifications in asthma provide self-management plans significantly more frequently than other nurses.

However a recent study in the BMJ showed that the concept of patient self-management plans received a lukewarm response from GPs, practice nurses and patients *(BMJ 2000;321:1507–10)*. Many patients are not actually interested in self-management plans; many believe they are already managing their asthma adequately! Asthma patients generally do not regard their condition as a chronic disease that needs regular monitoring and therapeutic adjustments, they prefer to manage it as an intermittent acute disorder.

What is the best way of identifying suboptimal control of asthma?
Although objective measurements of peak expiratory flow rate are important in assessing the severity and control of asthma, a symptom based assessment is also very useful in clinical practice *(BJGP 2000;50:7–12)*. The three best questions to use are:

Have you had difficulty sleeping because of your asthma?
Have you had your asthma symptoms during the day?
Has your asthma interfered with your usual activities?

Respiratory Diseases

 USEFUL WEBSITES

www.gpiag-asthma.org – GPs in asthma group
www.brit-thoracic.org.uk – British Thoracic Society

SUMMARY POINTS FOR ASTHMA

- ❖ BTS guidelines essential to learn
- ❖ CFC-free inhalers are replacing CFC inhalers
- ❖ NICE guidelines for childhood asthma are realistic
- ❖ Patients are not keen on self-management plans

Respiratory Diseases

CHRONIC OBSTRUCTIVE AIRWAYS DISEASE

In contrast to asthma, the BTS guidelines (published in 1997) on the management of patients with COAD have not had a huge impact on the management and are not a very successful guideline. They are also due to be reviewed soon. There is an emphasis on the use of spirometry to obtain objective evidence of both diagnosis and response to treatment.

Should spirometry be widely available in primary care?
This is an example of a 'pros and cons' type of question which often comes up in the exam.

Advantages	Disadvantages
• Convenient to patients	• Time and availability of staff to perform test
• Avoids waiting for appointment	• Cost of machinery and servicing
• Results readily available	• Lack of experience re interpretation of results
• Cheaper for NHS	• Lack of funding

Respiratory Diseases

SMOKING CESSATION

Smoking is the single greatest cause of preventable illness and premature death in the UK and leads to direct medical costs of £1.7 billion each year. Cigarette smoking will cause about 450 million deaths world-wide in the next 50 years. It is therefore a top healthcare priority, especially as there has been a recent increase in the number of smokers. The NHS Plan states that there will be a comprehensive smoking cessation service in place by 2001.

Around one in four adults smoke, with much higher levels in deprived sections of society. However, giving up permanently is difficult; although two-thirds of smokers want to quit, and about a third try each year, only 2% actually succeed.

On average, 70% of smokers consult their GP each year, so primary care teams need to be involved with smoking cessation programmes. The authors of the Sheffield table have even estimated that the statin bill could be reduced by 85% if everyone stopped smoking!

What are the updated smoking cessation guidelines?
In December 2000 Thorax published updated guidelines for tackling cigarette dependence *(Thorax 2000;55:987–99)*. They recognise that GPs have a pivotal role if the NHS is to deliver a noticeable drop in smoking rates. These guidelines are based on strong evidence from randomised trials supplemented by studies examining what can be achieved in routine clinical practice.

The guidelines recommend that all GPs give brief advice to all their patients who smoke at least once a year and if they respond positively they should then be referred to a smoking cessation clinic and considered for either nicotine replacement therapy or Zyban. GPs will therefore need to keep up-to-date records of patients' smoking status, advice they received and the response to that advice.

What are the advantages of stopping smoking?
There are obviously huge benefits from stopping smoking. Widespread cessation of smoking in the UK has already approximately halved the lung cancer mortality that would have been expected if former smokers had continued to smoke.

Underscoring the health benefits of smoking cessation is the report by Doll *et al.* based on a comparison of two case-control studies conducted 40 years apart in the UK *(BMJ 2000;321:323–9)*. Even smokers who stop at age 50 or 60 years avoid much of their excess risk of developing lung cancer. The benefits of cessation become progressively greater with younger age of quitting; stopping smoking before middle age avoids more than 90% of the risk attributable to tobacco.

How effective are smoking cessation treatments?

There is a wide array of effective smoking cessation treatments. A recent BMJ article provided an up to date and comprehensive review of the effectiveness of smoking cessation treatments *(BMJ 2000;321:355–8)*.

Nicotine Replacement Therapy (NRT)

This treatment aims to replace the nicotine obtained from cigarettes, thus reducing withdrawal symptoms when stopping smoking. Nicotine replacement is available as chewing gum, transdermal patch, nasal spray, inhaler, sublingual tablet and lozenge. A recent Cochrane review of over 90 trials found that nicotine replacement helps people to stop smoking. Overall, it increased the chances of quitting about one and a half to two times, whatever the level of additional support and encouragement. Since all the trials of nicotine replacement have included at least brief advice, this is the minimum that should be offered. More intensive support seems to be more effective; for example, NRT prescribed after GPs brief advice can result in up to 10% of smokers stopping but NRT together with support from specialist counsellors can result in up to 20% of smokers stopping.

There is little direct evidence that one nicotine product is more effective than another. Thus the decision about which product to use should be guided by individual preferences. Local arrangements may allow for a free supply of NRT to be made available to smokers attending for specialist treatment.

The government announced in April 2001 that it will allow NRT to be available on NHS prescriptions. Ministers plan to amend schedule 10 of NHS Regulations which lists items GPs may not prescribe. The decision fulfils the commitment the Government made in the NHS Plan. The Department of Health has estimated this will cost the NHS £10–40m.

Zyban (Bupropion)

This was initially developed as an antidepressant. One hypothesis of its mode of action is that it works by increasing levels of dopamine and noradrenaline in the brain, thereby counteracting the reductions in these chemicals that result from nicotine withdrawal. The efficacy of bupropion as an aid to smoking cessation has been investigated in two randomised, double-blinded, placebo-controlled trials *(NEMJ 1997; 337:1195–202, NEMJ 1999;340:685–91)*. These patients received regular counselling sessions in addition to bupropion. Results have indicated that up to 30% of smokers succeed with bupropion and these results are sustained over a year.

Zyban is relatively well tolerated; contraindications to it include epilepsy, pregnancy and concomitant antidepressants. The risk of fits has been estimated at about 1 in 1000 people which is actually the same risk as for amitriptyline and imipramine. Zyban may also increase the risk of fits through interactions with other drugs that lower the seizure threshold; including antipsychotics, antidepressants, systemic steroids, anti-malarial drugs and theophylline.

At least 420,000 patients have received Zyban since it was launched in the UK in June 2000. During this time there have been about 120 reports of seizures; approximately half of these occurred in patients who already had a history of seizures or were at risk of them. More concerning is that there has been a small number of deaths reported among people taking Zyban. These cases are currently being investigated further by the CSM; it is felt that in the majority of them the individual's underlying condition may actually have been the cause of death. The recommended dosage of Zyban was reduced in June 2001; the CSM has stated that the dose should be increased from day 7 of treatment rather than day 4.

It has been suggested that to prescribe Zyban, patients should answer yes to the following questions:
* Do you want to stop smoking?
* Is it very important for you to stop?
* Would you be prepared to stop smoking in the next two weeks?

Most patients are being prescribed Zyban in designated smoking cessation clinics where regular counselling and follow up can be provided, but this varies enormously across regions.

Other treatments
The effectiveness of other treatments, namely, aversion therapy, acupuncture, hypnotherapy and exercise is as yet uncertain.

What is the cycle of change and how can it be used for smoking cessation?

There are undoubtedly certain times when a patient will be more receptive to advice on stopping smoking. Smoking cessation should not be regarded as a dichotomous process (cessation or not) but rather as a continuum that entails several stages. DiClemente and Prochaska's cycle of readiness to change (see figure below) has been used to describe the psychological processes involved in many patterns of human behaviour and lends itself very well to smoking cessation (*J Consult Clin Psychol 1991;59:295–304*). It is important to know the 'cycle of change' as it can be applied to various aspects of clinical practice, and can be very useful to discuss in the viva examination!

DiClemente and Proschaska's cycle of change

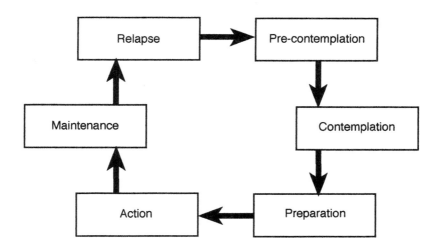

- **Precontemplation**

This is the stage at which the patient is happy at being a smoker and does not contemplate stopping. Although brief intervention at this stage may not persuade them to give up, it may help them question their habit and move them nearer to the next stage.

- **Contemplation**

This is the stage at which the patient is dissatisfied with being a smoker and is thinking about giving up (70% of adult smokers are at this stage!). During this stage, it can be effective to make the idea of quitting relevant to the patient, for example a patient recently diagnosed with heart disease.

- **Preparation**

This is the stage at which the smoker is making serious plans to stop. It is therefore important to be supportive and discussion about smoking cessation treatments is most beneficial at this stage.

- **Action**

This is the stage when maximum support should be given, as it is at this stage when the attempt to stop smoking is made.

- **Maintenance**

This is the stage at which the patient tries to prevent relapse. This is often the most difficult time as enthusiasm often wears off quicker than withdrawal symptoms.

- **Relapse**

This is obviously when the patient's attempt to stop smoking has been unsuccessful. This can either mean permanently giving up the idea of quitting smoking or thinking about it again in the future whereby the patient would then re-enter the cycle at the precontemplation stage once more.

If the doctor or health care professional is unaware of where their patient is in this cycle of change, then any time and effort given regarding smoking cessation may be wasted.

What is the role of doctors in smoking cessation?

Tobacco dependence is a chronic relapsing condition; like other addictions and chronic diseases, it warrants repeated clinical intervention. An important challenge is to integrate the available, evidence-based and cost-effective treatment of smoking cessation therapies into medical practice. The number of people successfully quitting smoking after using the smoking cessation services has actually been found to have more than doubled from April to September 2000 when compared with 1999.

In addition, by taking a few moments to identify where the patient is in the cycle of change, and tailoring the advice accordingly, the GP may be able to make each intervention more effective still.

Respiratory Diseases

🕸 USEFUL WEBSITES

www.update-software.com/ccweb/cochrane/revabstr/g160index.htm –
Cochrane reviews
www.nhs.uk/nhsplan – The NHS Plan

📋 SUMMARY POINTS FOR SMOKING CESSATION

- ❖ Over 75% smokers consult their GP annually
- ❖ Only 2% smokers manage to give up by themselves
- ❖ Smoking cessation clinics have promising results
- ❖ Zyban can help up to a third of smokers to stop smoking
- ❖ Assessing smokers' motivation to quit is important
- ❖ Consider the 'cycle of change'

41

Respiratory Diseases

INFLUENZA

During the winter months there is usually an outbreak of influenza, which results in a huge increase in workload for both primary care teams and hospitals. Even when the incidence is low, it has been estimated that 3–4000 deaths in the UK each year are from influenza-related causes.

What are the benefits of the influenza vaccine?
There is plenty of evidence to support the effectiveness of the vaccine; it reduces mortality and morbidity in high-risk groups. In May 2000 the policy on influenza vaccination was altered and the vaccine is now recommended for:
- All people over 65 years
- All people in long-stay residential accommodation
- All people with:
  - Chronic respiratory disease, including asthma
  - Chronic heart disease
  - Chronic renal disease
  - Diabetes mellitus
  - Immunosuppression due to disease or treatment

Various studies have demonstrated that the influenza vaccine can reduce mortality by around 40% compared with matched controls. For the first time, health authorities have been set a target of achieving a minimum of 65% uptake of immunisation in patients over 65 years.

A recent study showed a marked reduction in hospital admission for various diseases for people who had received the influenza vaccination *(Lancet 2001;357:1008–11)*. In particular there was a 46% reduction in admissions for influenza and a lower mortality from all causes (53–56% reduction).

When should Relenza be prescribed?
The National Institute for Clinical Excellence (NICE) recommended in November 2000 that zanamivir (Relenza) should be used to treat 'at risk' adults when influenza is circulating in the community and if they present within 36 hours of developing symptoms.

'At risk' adults are defined as those with:
- Chronic respiratory disease
- Significant cardiovascular disease
- Diabetes mellitus
- Age over 65 years

Respiratory Diseases

This recommendation reverses the Institute's ruling in 2000 that there was insufficient evidence of the drug's efficacy in high-risk individuals to make it worth prescribing on the NHS *(BMJ 1999;319:1024)*.

What is the evidence for Relenza?
Relenza is a neuraminidase antiviral compound which works by diminishing the replication of the influenza virus within host epithelial cells. It can be used for both influenza types A and B. The recommendations have been written following an overall pooled analysis of eight trials involving 800 adults at high risk and new research by GlaxoWellcome. The pooled analysis showed:
- Reduction in the duration of symptoms by 1.2 days (6 to 5 days)
- Reduction in duration of pyrexia by 1/2 day (2.5 to 2 days)
- 6% reduction in complications in which antibiotics were needed

When should Relenza be prescribed?
- If influenza has been shown to be circulating in the community
- Only to patients at high risk
- Within 36 hours of developing symptoms

Influenza is considered to be circulating in the community when consultations for influenza rise above 50 a week per 100,000 population, as monitored by the Royal College of General Practitioners' weekly returns monitoring service. The Public Health Laboratory Service must also have identified the circulation of an influenza virus.

Who will be responsible for prescribing Relenza?
These recommendations by NICE could potentially lead to a dramatic increase in GPs workload in the winter months. It has been suggested that pharmacists and nurses will be allowed to prescribe zanamivir under the generalised directions of a doctor, provided they are satisfied that the patient needs it and satisfies the criteria. Telephone triaging by practice nurses may also be set up; the nurses will work to a protocol and ask standard diagnostic questions. However, the question then arises regarding the person directly responsible for the patient if there is a complication from taking the drug; often this will be the patient's GP.

It has been estimated that 30% of self-diagnosed flu is actually due to influenza and as there is no cheap effective diagnostic test available. Many people may be unnecessarily prescribed or request Relenza.

Why is there opposition to prescribing Relenza?
The evidence to support Relenza is still from small studies and many of

Respiratory Diseases

the trials did not specifically recruit high-risk patients. Relenza's own product characteristics statement said it had been unable to determine that the drug was effective in elderly patients and those with chronic conditions such as asthma and diabetes. In addition there has been no published trial comparing Relenza's effect on influenza symptoms with symptomatic therapy (e.g. ibuprofen and paracetamol).

There have been reports of fatal adverse reactions in patients with COAD and asthma in the USA. It has therefore been recommended that if Relenza is to be prescribed for patients with airways disease, it should be done only under careful supervision with short-acting bronchodilators available. Any persuasive evidence of Relenza's cost-effectiveness is still lacking – NICE's own guidance states 'no reliable data are available as to the impact on the use of Relenza on hospitalisation or mortality'.

NICE originally refused to allow the drug to be prescribed on the NHS last year and the BMJ has criticised NICE for responding to 'political clout'. Drugs and Therapeutics Bulletin will still continue not to recommend Relenza as part of treatment of influenza as it is 'unconvinced of the benefits'.

Finally, a recent study has found that most elderly people can not actually use the inhaler device correctly *(BMJ 2001;322:577–9)*. One of the authors of the study has advised that GPs need to spend at least 15 minutes teaching their elderly patients how to use the device; this is not really realistic.

 USEFUL WEBSITES

www.phls.co.uk/facts/influenza/flu.htm – Up-to-date information from the Public Health Laboratory Service
www.rcgp-bru.demon.co.uk – Influenza surveillance website
www.nice.org.uk – NICE guidelines
Obesity is rapidly becoming a major threat to health. The prevalence of

---

SUMMARY POINTS FOR INFLUENZA

- ❖ Influenza leads to about 3,000 deaths annually
- ❖ Influenza vaccine is safe and effective
- ❖ NICE recommends use of Relenza
- ❖ Weak evidence to support Relenza

CHAPTER 3: OBESITY

obesity (defined as a body mass index >30 kg/m^2) in the UK is increasing; by 2005 it has been estimated that 18% men and 25% women will be obese. In addition, reports suggest that the prevalence of obesity among children is also increasing – presently 1 in 5 9-year-olds and 1 in 3 11-year-old girls are overweight. More people now die prematurely from obesity related conditions than road traffic accidents in the UK!

What are the problems with obesity?
Obesity results in a huge financial burden to healthcare. It is a significant aetiological factor in many common diseases. These include diabetes, hypertension, hyperlipidaemia, ischaemic heart disease and stroke. Obesity is associated with increased mortality, particularly from cardiovascular disease *(NEMJ 1999; 341:1097–105)*. The medical costs of obesity have been estimated to account for 5–8% of all healthcare expenditure.

The National Audit Office published a report in February 2001 entitled 'Tackling Obesity in England' which stated that national guidelines should be produced on the management of overweight and obese patients in primary care.

What are the benefits of a modest weight reduction?
For many obese people, achieving their ideal body weight is unrealistic and impossible. However, significant benefits can be gained from even a 10% loss of body weight, which is more achievable and sustainable. These benefits include a reduction in blood pressure, reduction in total cholesterol (including rise in HDL cholesterol) and reduced risk of developing diabetes.

What drugs are available to treat obesity?
Many of the drugs that have been used in the past were centrally acting appetite suppressants, which are either addictive or associated with pulmonary hypertension and valvular heart disease, so are not now used.

Orlistat
Orlistat is an intestinal lipase inhibitor that blocks the absorption of about 30% of dietary fat. In clinical trials of up to two years duration it resulted in an average weight loss of about 10%, compared with 6% in the placebo group *(Lancet 1998;352:167–72)*. There is good evidence to

Obesity

support its effect on weight reduction both in the short-term and 1–2 years post treatment. Other benefits of Orlistat include reduction in LDL and total cholesterol, a reduction in blood pressure and improvements in insulin resistance and blood glucose control in diabetic patients. A study of Orlistat in patients with non-insulin diabetes mellitus demonstrated that 43% patients reduced their sulphonylurea dose and 12% patients actually stopped their oral diabetic medication.

The licensing criteria for the drug require patients to lose at least 2.5 kg in four weeks prior to starting treatment and they should only continue with the drug if they achieve a weight loss of at least a further 5% of their body weight after the first 12 weeks of treatment and a cumulative weight loss of at least 10% after the first six months.

NICE has recently produced guidance on the use of Orlistat and have agreed it can be prescribed as long as doctors stick to the strict conditions of its product licence and it is only used for patients who are either clinically obese or are overweight (BMI $\geq$ 28 kg/m^2) with other health-related problems (such as Type 2 diabetes or hypertension).

Roche, who produce Orlistat, have provided a freephone number (0800 731 7138) so patients are registered and given dietary and lifestyle advice. They are also contacted regularly to provide additional support and encouragement, which seems to be very beneficial.

What is Reductil?
Another new anti-obesity drug, Reductil (sibutramine), became available in June 2001. The recently published STORM (sibutramine trial of obesity reduction and maintenance) trial differs from other weight loss trials as its objective was to test whether treatment with Reductil could prevent weight regain among patients who had already achieved a weight loss of more than 5% of their body weight *(Lancet 2000;356:2119–25)*. The study showed that 43% of the patients treated with Reductil maintained at least 80% of their body weight loss compared with only 16% in the placebo group. In addition, significant changes in cardiovascular disease risk factors were noted, including reduced triglyceride concentrations, increased HDL-cholesterol concentrations and reduced cholesterol:HDL-cholesterol ratio.

Reductil works by inhibiting the re-uptake of the neurotransmitters noradrenaline and serotonin, thereby leading to increased feelings of satiety after eating. The UK licence for Reductil specifies a maximum

Obesity

treatment period of 12 months and has similar constraints to use as Orlistat. It is contraindicated in patients with coronary heart disease, peripheral vascular disease and inadequately controlled hypertension or hyperthyroidism.

 USEFUL WEBSITES

www.nice.org.uk – NICE guidelines
www.nao.gov.uk/publications/nao_reports/index.htm – 'Tackling Obesity on England' report

---

SUMMARY POINTS FOR OBESITY

- ❖ Prevalence of obesity dramatically increasing
- ❖ Obesity is huge financial burden to healthcare
- ❖ Numerous benefits gained from losing small amounts of weight
- ❖ Orlistat has been approved by NICE

CHAPTER 4: PSYCHIATRY

MENTAL HEALTH NATIONAL SERVICE FRAMEWORK

The Mental Health National Service Framework was announced in October 1999. It was initially proposed in 1998 in the white paper '*A first class service: quality in the new NHS*', and was proposed as an *accompaniment* to NICE. The framework sets national standards for mental health services and is based on clinical evidence. It sets out best practice for promoting mental health and treating mental illness. It comes with an extra £700m for mental health services over the next three years and aims to iron out unacceptable variations around the country. There are plans to integrate health and social services.

Seven standards of care

1. Combat discrimination against people with mental health problems
2. Identification of needs and adequate assessment – patients offered appropriate treatment or referral
3. 24-hour availability of services for mental health patients
4. Written care plans
5. Provide beds in a secure, protective environment close to home service users who need a 'period of care' away from home. Patients should have timely access to an appropriate bed, which should be close to home and in the least restrictive environment consistent with the need to protect them and the public.
6. Assess the needs of the carer
7. Reduce suicide by implementing the above and develop local systems for suicide audit

Criticisms of the Mental Health National Service Framework
* Long overdue – too little, too late
* Laudable aims
* Government branding and propaganda
* Is money enough when underfunded for 20 years?
* 24-hour access – is NHS Direct enough?
* 'Evidence' quoted is very subjective - how can you audit discrimination?

Psychiatry

 Reforming the Mental Health Act (December 2000)

This White Paper sets out the Government's plans for new mental health legislation. It will:
- Form part of new arrangements for improving the quality and consistency of health and social care services for the many people who suffer from mental health problems
- Provide a new structure for the application of compulsory powers of detention for assessment and treatment (previously termed 'sections') for the small minority of those who pose a serious threat to the safety of others as a result of their mental disorder

New mental health legislation will provide a single framework for the application of compulsory powers for care and treatment. This will include:
- Common criteria
- Common pathway for assessment
- Approval of a plan of care and treatment by the Mental Health Tribunal
- An improved and more consistent set of safeguards for all patients

There are two parts to this White Paper. This is to distinguish arrangements for high risk group patients.

Reforms are a response to
- Media publicity regarding dangerous and severely personality disordered (DSPD) patients and the tragic toll of homicides and suicides
- Public confidence in care in the community has been undermined by failures in services and failures in the law
- Current 1983 Mental Health Act is largely based on a review of mental health legislation which took place in the 1950s, outmoded laws have failed to protect the public, patients or staff properly
- Under existing mental health laws, the powers for compulsory treatment are for patients in hospital only, whilst the majority of patients today are treated in the community
- Severely ill patients have been allowed to drift out of contact with mental health services and have been able to refuse treatment
- Existing legislation has also failed to provide adequate public protection from those whose risk to others arises from a severe personality disorder

Psychiatry

Of course the vast majority of people with mental illness represent no threat to anyone. Many mentally ill patients are among the most vulnerable members of society. But the Government has a duty to protect individual patients and the public, if a person poses a serious risk to themselves or to others.

PART 1 – SUMMARY

- Improving the quality and consistency of health and social care services
- Extra investment in services and national standards of care by April 2001, almost 500 extra secure beds, over 320 24-hour staffed beds, 170 assertive outreach teams and access to services 24 hours a day, seven days a week, for all those with complex mental health needs
- The *NHS Plan* announced a further £300m investment to provide better and faster care to people with mental health problems who need treatment and support, including new services for children and adolescents
- New national standards for the care and treatment of mental illness in the *Mental Health NSF*
- More effective and accessible community based support
- Principles of common law do not always provide the sort of robust framework that is needed to protect people from the effects of serious mental disorder and to enable action necessary to prevent serious harm
- Government has a duty to set out a clear framework in mental health legislation for determining when and how care and treatment for mental disorder may be provided without consent in the best interests of a patient or to prevent serious harm to other people

Areas discussed in Part 1

Safeguarding human rights
- Includes powers to place significant restrictions on the personal liberty of patients, in particular the freedom to refuse care and treatment
- New mental health legislation must be fully compatible with the Human Rights Act 1998
- Revised broad definition of mental disorder covering any disability or disorder of mind or brain, whether permanent or temporary,

50

which results in an impairment or disturbance of mental functioning
- Matched by criteria that set clear limits to the circumstances in which compulsory powers may be used
- Diagnosis of mental disorder alone would never be sufficient to justify use of compulsory powers
- Use of compulsory powers will generally only be appropriate if a person is resisting care and treatment needed either in their best interests or because without care and treatment they will pose a significant risk of serious harm to other people
- Sets out what should be covered in the care and treatment plan

New safeguards
- New independent tribunal to determine all longer-term use of compulsory powers
- New right to independent advocacy
- New safeguards for people with long-term mental incapacity
- New Commission for Mental Health
- Statutory requirement to develop care plans

New procedures for use of compulsory powers
New three-stage process that applies in all cases, except for offenders (for whom assessment will be ordered by the Court) and for prisoners (the Home Secretary):

Stage 1 – Preliminary examination
- When a patient needs further assessment or urgent treatment by specialist mental health services and, without this, might be at risk of serious harm or pose a risk of serious harm to other people
- Decisions to begin assessment and initial treatment of a patient under compulsory powers will be based on a preliminary examination by two doctors and a social worker or another suitably trained mental health professional

Stage 2 – Formal assessment and initial treatment under compulsory powers
- Patients will be given a full assessment of their health and social care needs and receive treatment set out in a formal care plan
- Initial period of assessment and treatment under compulsory powers will be limited to a maximum of 28 days
- After that, continuing use of compulsory powers must be authorised by a new independent decision-making body, the

Psychiatry

Mental Health Tribunal, which will obtain advice from independent experts as well as taking evidence from the clinical team, the patient and his or her representatives and other agencies, where appropriate

Stage 3 – Care and treatment order

- The Tribunal (or Court in the case of mentally disordered offenders) will be able to make a care and treatment order which will authorise the care and treatment specified in a care plan recommended by the clinical team.
- This must be designed to give therapeutic benefit to the patient or to manage behaviour associated with mental disorder that might lead to serious harm to other people.
- The first two orders will be for up to 6 months each; subsequent orders may be for periods of up to 12 months.

Care and treatment in the community

- Introduce new provisions so that care and treatment orders may apply to patients outside hospital
- Will mean that patients need not be in hospital unnecessarily and need not suffer the possible distress of repeated unplanned admissions to acute wards
- Will be no powers for patients to be given medication forcibly **except** in a clinical setting
- Steps will be specified in community orders to prevent patients, if they do not comply with their order, becoming a risk to themselves, their carers, or the public
- New legislation will also introduce a new duty covering the disclosure of information about patients suffering from mental disorder between health and social services agencies and other agencies (e.g. housing agencies or criminal justice agencies)

Better information and advice

- Every patient will be informed about the particular powers that apply in his or her case
- Patients who want to challenge the use of compulsory powers will continue to have the right to free legal representation
- Will also give them a new right of access to advice and support from independent specialist advocacy services – 'The new Patient Advocacy Liaison Service' (PALS)

Psychiatry

New safeguards for children and young people
- Mental Health Tribunal will be required to obtain specialist expert advice on both health and social care aspects of the proposed care plan and to consider whether the location of care is appropriate
- Decisions taken in respect of children will be subject to a clear principle that the interests of the child must be paramount
- Changes in the provisions regarding the right of a young person between the ages of 16 and 18 to refuse consent to care and treatment for mental disorder

New safeguards for people with long-term mental incapacity
- Potentially vulnerable to abuse or neglect, must ensure that their best interests are properly considered and protected
- Can only be achieved through an independent consideration of the care that they receive for their mental disorder
- Place a duty on the clinical supervisor responsible for the care and treatment of a patient with long-term mental incapacity to carry out an assessment and obtain an independent second opinion

A new Commission for Mental Health
- To look after the interests of all people who are subject to care and treatment under powers in the Act
- Will carry specific responsibilities for monitoring the use of formal powers, providing guidance on the operation of those powers, and assuring the quality of statutory training provided for practitioners with key responsibilities under the new legislation and for specialist advocacy services

PART 2 – HIGH RISK PATIENTS
- Patients who pose a significant risk of serious harm to others
- Vast majority of people treated under mental health legislation are treated in their own best interests, in many cases to protect them from self-harm
- By contrast, there are a smaller number of people with a mental disorder who are characterised by the risk that they present to others
- This group includes a very small number of people detained under civil powers and others who are remanded or convicted offenders
- Within this wider group are a number of individuals whose risk is as a result of a severe personality disorder

Psychiatry

A narrow interpretation of the definition of the 'treatability' provision in the 1983 Act, together with a lack of dedicated provision within existing services, means that current arrangements for this group are inadequate both to protect the public and to provide the individuals themselves with the high quality services they need.

The criteria
- New criteria for compulsory treatment under the Act will form a key part of these changes
- Deal separately with those who need treatment primarily in their own best interests and those who need treatment because of the risk that they pose to others
- In high-risk cases, the use of compulsory powers will be linked to the availability of a treatment plan needed either to **treat** the underlying mental disorder or to **manage behaviours** arising from the disorder

Powers in the Criminal Justice and Court Services Act 2000, expected to be implemented in April 2001, will mean that the police and probation services will be under a new statutory duty to assess and manage relevant sexual or violent offenders.

Under new mental health legislation, the relevant statutory agencies will be able to refer the individual for an initial assessment and, if the initial criteria are satisfied, apply for a 28 day period of compulsory care and treatment to allow for more detailed assessment.

Beyond 28 days, compulsory care must be authorised by the new 'Mental Health Tribunal'.

In addition to existing facilities, assessment facilities for those who are 'dangerous and severely personality disordered' (DSPD) are being established for the in-depth assessment needed for this group.

Treatment
Under new legislation, the Tribunal (or Court for offenders) will be able to make a care and treatment order which will authorise the care and treatment specified in a care plan recommended by the clinical team. The first two orders will be for up to 6 months each; subsequent orders may be for periods of up to 12 months. Where treatment is authorised under the legislation, individuals will be transferred to appropriate NHS facilities taking account of any security risks that they pose. Wherever

54

Psychiatry

possible, treatment will be specifically aimed at addressing the underlying mental disorder. But in all high risk cases, treatment will be designed both to manage the consequences of a mental disorder as well as to enable the individuals themselves to work towards successful re-integration into the community.

Are these to be the modern day asylums?

Safeguards
All those detained under compulsory powers will also have the right to:
- Free legal representation
- Access to independent specialist advocacy services
- Provisions to cover the use of certain specified treatments for mental disorder and all long-term treatment without consent

Developing services for the DSPD
Recent spending review across the DoH, Home Office and Prison Service includes an additional £126m over the next three years for the development of new specialist services for those who are high risk as a result of a severe personality disorder.

- Committed to a series of pilot projects to test out new approaches
- Assessment process is already being piloted in both NHS and Prison Service high security settings and the first treatment pilot will begin in 2001
- Over the next three years this will provide
  – an extra 320 specialist places across HMP/NHS
  – an extra 75 hostel places
- Introduction of new arrangements for the provision of information to victims of mentally disordered offenders who have committed serious violent or sexual offences and who have been given a care and treatment order by the Courts rather than a prison sentence

The full document can be found on the internet:

 www.doh.gov.uk/mentalhealth

Psychiatry

DEPRESSION

A popular topic which always appears in the exam.

- Common: 10–15% of people suffer a significant depressive illness
- Under-diagnosed: about 50% of depression is missed
- Under treated: antidepressants are effective with a NNT of 3

Detection
Evidence shows good levels of concordance between GP diagnosis of depression and DSM IV diagnosis, using these criteria could increase GPs diagnostic sensitivity.

DSM IV criteria (simplified):
Over the last two weeks, five of the following features should be present for a diagnosis of major depression, of which one or more should be

- Depressed mood
- Anhedonia - loss of interest or pleasure

And the remaining to make a total of 5:
- Significant change in weight or appetite
- Change in sleep
- Psychomotor agitation or retardation
- Fatigue/loss of energy
- Feelings of worthlessness/guilt
- Loss of concentration
- Recurrent thoughts of death/suicidal ideas

Useful as some patients with an acute episode may appear low in mood, tearful and appear highly distressed but they do not meet these criteria and there is less evidence that they are helped by antidepressants.
For some with a chronic depressive disorder (dysthymia) who do not meet DSM IV there is some evidence that drugs may help (possibly short-term).

PAPERS:

 Hampshire Depression Project (HDP)
(Lancet 2000;355:185)

- Large well designed RCT of teaching practitioners about the recognition and management of depression and using patient improvement as the outcome measure
- RCT that gave 4 hours education to GPs – tailored to their needs and nothing to the controls
- 22,000 people were screened using a standardised protocol
- Sensitivity of detection was 36% in the control group and 39% in the education group
- Results disappointingly negative, failing to show any increase in recognition or patient recovery rates
- Casts doubt on the claim that detection is improved with education and was open to criticism from GPs and psychiatrists alike
- In an editorial *(Lancet)* GPs were accused of not following guidelines

Shortly afterwards an editorial entitled 'Why can't GPs follow guidelines on depression?' appeared in the *BMJ* discussing the issues raised by the study *(BMJ 2000;320:200)*.

Issues discussed and points raised:

- Findings of the HDP herald the need for a major change in thinking about improving the management of depression in primary care
- Results conflict with the positive findings of other studies (note the HDP had more participants)
- Such intensive training as used in the HDP cannot be delivered through our existing education systems

A review of 45 guidelines for depression showed they all have three common recommendations:
- Practitioners seek cases of 'major depressive disorder'
- Treatment is advised if patients have enough symptoms for long enough (even if social causes are identified)
- Most recommend tricyclics (TCA) as first-line treatment (in dose equivalents of 125 mg/day of amitriptyline and continuing for four months after recovery)

Problems exist with these recommendations:
- Diagnosis is not easy to make in primary care, symptoms change quickly, cut off levels for duration are somewhat arbitrary
- Practitioners vary significantly in the threshold at which they treat. Many practitioners doubt the effectiveness of antidepressants in the face of social problems. Guidelines are based on a RCT of amitriptyline versus placebo, patients with 'major' depression responded whilst those with minor depression did not, irrespective of whether the depression was endogenous or non-endogenous (i.e. attributed to social problems). Other research shows social factors in the short-term are associated with persistence of depression.
- Patients are often reluctant to accept drugs. Much of the public believe that depression is due to adverse life events and that counselling should be offered. Most think that antidepressants are addictive. Explains why patients take sub-therapeutic doses of tricyclics and discontinue early. Advent of SSRIs has increased the proportion taking therapeutic doses, but still do not continue treatment for the recommended duration.

May explain why recognition of depression and subsequent drug treatment in primary care is not associated with better outcomes. The author states the '...negative findings of the HDP must be viewed in this context.' The effectiveness of SSRIs for minor depression has not been established in primary care. Neither has effectiveness of counselling been wholly validated.

 Antidepressant drugs and generic counselling for treatment of major depression in primary care.
(BMJ 2001;322:772).

- Objective was to compare the efficacy of antidepressant drugs and generic counselling for treating mild to moderate depression in general practice
- RCT with patient preference arms (i.e. allowed to choose rather than be randomised), followed up at 8 weeks and 12 months
- 31 General Practices in Trent region with 103 patients randomised and 220 patients in preference arms
- Study looked at the Beck depression inventory score (validated), time to remission and global outcome assessed by a psychiatrist

Conclusions
- Statistical tests showed no significant differences in effectiveness so authors state generic counselling seems to be as effective as antidepressants for mild to moderate depressive illness
- Patients receiving antidepressants may recover more quickly
- GPs should allow patients to have their preferred treatment 12 months after starting treatment, generic counselling is as effective as antidepressants
- Patients who choose counselling may benefit more than those with no strong preference

Criticisms
- Data interpretation should be regarded with caution due to small sample sizes and difficulties in follow up
- Study placed few constraints on either the drug treatment or the type of counselling other than that the counselling should be provided by an experienced mental health professional in six sessions
- Therefore compared non-standardised antidepressant use with non-standardised counselling by experienced professionals

Modern Drug Treatment of Depression.
(BMJ 1999;318:1188–91). Used in Clinical Evidence 2000.

- All have 50–60% improvement
- 30–40% on placebo
- Anecdote strongly favours SSRIs in terms of tolerability
- SSRIs are 30 times more expensive than tricyclics, cost effectiveness has not been established as a first-line treatment
- Certain groups likely to benefit: the elderly; those at risk of suicide; those with cardiac or prostatic symptoms
- 4–6 months drug therapy is advocated after the initial treatment phase to prevent relapse
- Trial of 6 weeks should be carried out before giving up
- If second-line is needed, use another class
- Stopping SSRIs, tail off over 4 weeks. SSRIs with a short half-life (paroxetine) have greater discontinuation reactions than those with long half-lives (fluoxetine).

Psychiatry

 Evaluation of a mental health facilitator in General Practice.
(BMJ 2000;50:626)

- Looked at the role of a mental health facilitator in General Practice
- Already shown to improve GP management in stroke, heart disease and asthma
- Aims to:
1. Form a relationship with the PHCT
2. Encourage assessment of current practice
3. Offer resources to assist process of change (e.g. guidelines)
4. Promote teamwork in the PHCT and improve links with secondary care providers
5. Organise educational activity
- Study was a RCT of 6 practices with facilitators and 6 controls.

Conclusions
- Improved recognition of mental illness
- No fundamental change in treatment and outcome
- As usual authors stated further development is needed

 The effectiveness of exercise as an intervention in the management of depression.
(BMJ 2001;322:763)

- Systematic review of RCTs to determine the effectiveness of exercise as an intervention in the management of depression
- Analysis was difficult as all studies were methodologically flawed
- How do you 'blind' treatment in which you have to partake?
- Difficult to separate the fact that people may interact socially when they exercise and that this may act as a benefit
- No apparent difference existed between aerobic or non-aerobic exercise
- Concluded effectiveness of exercise in reducing symptoms of depression cannot be determined because of a lack of good quality research with adequate follow up and that as usual, a well designed RCT is needed
- Does this mean that 'exercise on prescription' for depression is futile or do you carry on funding beneficial social interaction and hope for some health promotion?

Psychiatry

Use of St John's Wort in Depression
- Hippocrates described the use of *Hypericum perforatum* (St John's Wort) as a treatment against demonic possession in ancient Greece
- Used extensively as first-line treatment for depression and anxiety in Germany
- Widespread use (2 million in UK)
- Meta-analysis showed it is effective compared with placebo, NNT of 4 over 4 weeks of treatment *(BMJ 1996;313:253)*
- RCT compared 350 mg St John's Wort tds/100 mg of imipramine/placebo – TCA and St John's Wort had an equal therapeutic response, side-effects were the same as for placebo *(BMJ 1999;319:1534)*
- A further German RCT *(BMJ 2000;321:536)* compared 75 mg bd imipramine with 250 mg St John's Wort for 6 weeks in outpatients; found that it was therapeutically equivalent to imipramine in treating mild to moderate depression, but patients tolerate St John's Wort better.
- St John's Wort can induce liver enzymes
- Drug interactions with digoxin, theophylline, warfarin and COCP (CSM warning March 2000)

See page 181 for further information on St John's Wort.

61

Psychiatry

POST-NATAL DEPRESSION (DTB May 2000)

- Common
- Little evidence for aetiology; antenatal, personal and social factors more relevant
- 10–15% of deliveries
- Many recover spontaneously
- 50% still depressed at 6 months
- 33% go on to develop a chronic, recurrent mood disorder
- Associated with disturbances in the mother-infant relationship, which in turn has an adverse impact on child cognitive and emotional development
- Must distinguish between common maternity 'blues' (= emotional lability, peak day 3–5, over by day 10)
- Depression more likely if previous psychiatric/family history, social problems, bereavement
- Poor detection
- Detection rates are improved by routine use of The Edinburgh Post-natal Depression Score (validated detection tool)
- Treatment:
  - Counselling (HV/GP)
  - CBT
  - Antidepressants all effective (SSRI/TCA appear to be safe with breast feeding)
  - Refer if psychotic/suicidal (mother and baby unit)

SCHIZOPHRENIA

 How to Manage the First Episode of Schizophrenia
(BMJ 2000;321:522–3)

- 1% lifetime prevalence
- GP will have 4–8/2000 patients
- Increasing evidence that the early stages of the disease are critical in forming and predicting the course and outcome of the disease
- Early treatment may result in a better prognosis and functional outcome
- Patients have the disease for 2–3 years before a diagnosis is made
- Early diagnosis is difficult due to insidious nature of the condition
- Prevalence of pre-morbid problems in language/cognitive ability/drug use etc
- Editorial suggests a reluctance to make an early diagnosis - wasting a therapeutic window of opportunity

We need to

- Make the diagnosis early
- Look for 'negative' symptoms (emotional flattening, poor motivation, anhedonia and loss of self care) plus positive symptoms (auditory hallucinations, delusions and thought disorder)
- Provide effective treatment with multi-disciplinary teams
- Drugs used to control symptoms – use those that minimise side-effects as a first-line to maximise long-term compliance
- 70% of people after a first attack will relapse within 5 years, so early drug withdrawal is not recommended. If poor clinical response, second-line drugs such as clozapine should be used early.
- After acute phase – intensive community rehabilitation, family therapy, CBT all improve long-term social functioning.

Psychiatry

THE NEW ANTI-PSYCHOTIC DRUGS

Reviewed **BJGP** *(RCGP;49:745–9)*

- Pimozide/clozapine are useful in patients who have not responded to current drugs
- They have potentially serious side-effects and need close monitoring
- Conflicting evidence as to whether the newer drugs are more beneficial on the 'negative' symptoms of schizophrenia
- Open minded and hopeful about their effects
- There are purchasing difficulties

Clinical Evidence 2000 quotes systematic reviews showing:
- Equal efficacy of olanzapine and risperidone with standard anti-psychotics but reduced side-effects
- Clear evidence of benefit of clozapine in people resistant to standard treatment
- Lower relapse rates with prolonged maintenance treatment (up to 2 years)
- Lower relapse rates with clozapine
- Clear evidence that social interventions such as family therapy significantly reduce relapse rates

 Atypical anti-psychotics, patients value the lower incidence of extrapyramidal side-effects.
(BMJ 2000;321:1360)

This editorial appeared in the BMJ alongside a systematic review of atypicals, points raised were:
- No clinically significant evidence of superiority in efficacy, or for that matter tolerability, for atypical antipsychotics as a group
- Atypical antipsychotics account for nearly three out of four new prescriptions for antipsychotics in North America
- Atypicals have a lower incidence of extrapyramidal side-effects
- Extrapyramidal side-effects are not just incidental 'side' effects but the central factor in many patients agendas
- Extrapyramidal effects by themselves have been related to a poor outcome, a compromised compliance, secondary negative symptoms, cognitive parkinsonism and depression as well as long-term risk of tardive dyskinesia
- May turn out that the real superiority of atypicals is not in their

Psychiatry

antipsychotic abilities but in their ability to control ancillary symptoms related to mood, cognition, hostility and a higher level of compliance
- Atypical agents have their own new side-effects such as weight gain and diabetes

This is a case where efficiency alone cannot constitute good treatment.

Psychiatry

EATING DISORDERS

Always think of the possibility of an eating disorder as a 'hidden agenda'. It may be the underlying problem when patients present with tiredness, aches and pains as well as irritable bowel and amenorrhoea. Some patients may have alexithymia, this is a difficulty in identifying and expressing emotion and in distinguishing between emotions and somatic sensation. Rates: 1:2000 anorexia, 20:2000 bulimia, 40:2000 'partial' syndromes. Treatments include CBT, SSRIs. Early intervention produces better outcome.

Diagnostic criteria for anorexia nervosa
- Over-concern with shape and weight, with intense fear of becoming fat
- Active maintenance of low weight (body mass index <17.5) by strict dieting, excessive exercising and possibly self-induced vomiting
- Amenorrhoea for a minimum of three months (if not taking the COCP)

Diagnostic criteria for bulimia nervosa
- Characteristic over-concern with shape and weight
- Frequent binges (bulimic episodes)
- Extreme behaviour to prevent weight gain (self-induced vomiting, purgative and diuretic abuse, fasting)

Binge eating
Eating in a period of time an amount of food that is larger than most people would eat in a similar period/situation. May have a sense of lack of control.

Atypical eating disorders
Disorders that do not fulfil the above criteria (i.e. binge eating without extreme weight controlling behaviour).

Psychiatry

📖 *The SCOFF questionnaire: assessment of a new screening tool for eating disorders.*
(BMJ 1999;319:1467)

Enables non-specialists to make a rapid assessment as to whether or not an eating disorder was likely.

1. Do you ever make yourself **S**ick because you feel uncomfortably full?
2. Do you ever worry you have lost **C**ontrol over how much you eat?
3. Have you ever lost more than **O**ne stone over a one month period?
4. Do you believe yourself to be **F**at when others say you are thin?
5. Would you say **F**ood dominates your life?

*   Each yes scores one point
*   When compared with lengthy detailed questionnaires to evaluate the test you get these results
*   Threshold of diagnosis is 2 or greater, gives a sensitivity of 100% for anorexia and bulimia separately and combined
*   Specificity of 87.5%
*   Only 12.5% false positive rate

ALCOHOL

Safe Limit (Government figures) 21 units per week for women and 28 units for men. Lowest mortality is achieved by drinking between 7 and 21 units a week. 45:2000 patients will be physically dependent.

Two approaches to tackle the problem:

- High Risk Approach   Target small group of heavy drinkers.
- Population approach   Aim is to reduce average alcohol consumption so that a general reduction in consumption will also reduce the numbers of problem drinkers (DoH estimates 1% increase in the price leads to 1% reduction in consumption).

The CAGE questionnaire

Have you ever felt you should **C**ut down on your drinking?
Have people ever **A**nnoyed you by criticising your drinking?
Have you ever felt **G**uilty about your drinking?
Have you ever had to have a drink first thing in the morning to steady your nerves or to get rid of a hangover (**E**ye opener)?

If answer yes to 2 or more then there is an 80–90% chance that a drinking problem exists.

 Alcohol consumption and mortality from all causes, coronary heart disease and stroke: results from a prospective cohort study of Scottish men with 21 years of follow up.
(BMJ 1999;318:1725)

- 5766 men aged 35–64 when screened in 1970–3 who answered questions on their usual weekly alcohol consumption
- Aim was to define mortality from all causes, coronary heart disease, stroke and alcohol related causes over 21 years of follow up related to units of alcohol consumed per week
- Risk for all cause mortality was similar for non-drinkers and men drinking up to 14 units/week
- Mortality risk then showed a graded association with alcohol consumption

Psychiatry

- No strong relation between alcohol consumption and mortality from coronary heart disease
- Strong positive relationship between alcohol and risk of mortality from stroke
- Men drinking 35 or more units have double the risk of stroke compared with non-drinkers
- No clear evidence of any protective effect for men drinking <22 units/week
- Different relations between alcohol consumption and mortality than previous studies
- Some but not all of this could be accounted for by alcohol-related increases in blood pressure
- Overall, risk of all cause mortality was higher in men drinking ≥22 units/week

Psychiatry

DRUGS

50% of young people have consumed an illegal drug. Poverty, inequality and social exclusion contribute to serious drug problems. 60% of people arrested test positive for illegal drugs (20% for opiates). There is an increasing problem of drugs and RTAs.

Guidelines on Clinical Management, Department of Health 1999
- Drug misusers have the same entitlement to NHS provisions as anyone else
- Doctors to provide care for general health and drug related problems (e.g. Hep B)
- Importance of a shared care approach
- Doctors not to be pressurised into accepting responsibility beyond their level of skill
- Support should include expert clinical advice and guidance on medico-legal matters
- Prescription is an enhancement to other psychological, social and medical interventions
- Ensuring that there is clear evidence of dependence/ withdrawal/ tolerance before treatment
- Supervised consumption advised for the first 3 months, continue if there are any doubts about compliance
- Evidence exists that maintenance treatment can enable patients to achieve stability
- Doctors responsibility to ensure that the patient receives the correct dose
- Doctors responsibility to ensure that drugs are not diverted to other users
- Prescribing of tablets and injectables strongly discouraged
- Stop short of recommending diamorphine prescribing despite evidence

Criticisms
- Doctor's reservations
- Funding
- Time (supervision in a problem area: 100+ people per day)
- Controversial view that time spent would lead to reduction in services elsewhere

Psychiatry

Cannabis trial launched in patients with multiple sclerosis
The world's biggest clinical trial of the cannabis plant started in January 2001 at Derriford Hospital, Plymouth.

- Looking at the control of pain and tremors in multiple sclerosis
- The cannabis in multiple sclerosis (CAMS) study is sponsored by the Medical Research Council
- Approved by the Government, which has arranged for the drug to be imported from Switzerland
- A parallel study will examine the effect of the drug on lower urinary tract symptoms
- Cannabis has been a schedule 1 drug since 1971, when the WHO pronounced it medically useless
- Two years ago a House of Lords select committee argued that more research was necessary in view of reports of the drug's efficacy in controlling pain and tremor in multiple sclerosis

Psychiatry

COUNSELLING

Q. *What is counselling?*
A. *It is helping patients to identify, understand, come to terms and cope with their problems.*

Skills needed for counselling

Listening	Summarising
Empathising	Interpreting
Reflecting	Confronting
Clarifying	Motivating

Various counselling styles

• Directive	Counsellor acts prescriptively
• Informative	Counsellor provides information to help decision-making
• Confrontational	Counsellor challenges unhelpful thinking/behaviour
• Cathartic	Counsellor encourages expression of hidden thoughts/fears/guilt
• Catalytic	Counsellor encourages patient to establish own goals/take control
• Supportive	Counsellor provides acceptance, empathy, concern for patient's anxieties and needs
• Rogerian	Counsellor provides non-directive listening rather than advice, encouraging patient to make decisions based on own judgement

Who does it?

GP	Uses counselling skills usually in course of normal surgery
Attached counsellor	Longer interviews with protected time
	Need to ensure competence
	Need to ensure integration in PHCT

Does it work?

Evidence suggests counselling in General Practice is an effective therapy for psychosocial problems and minor affective disorders.

Psychiatry

Some trials (not all) show that doctors
- Identify more problems
- Prescribe fewer drugs
- Investigate less
- Refer less

Patients
- Get relief from symptoms
- Cope better with feelings
- Cope better with life
- Consult less often

More information is needed on value of types of counselling and skills of counsellors.

What is the case against?
- Doctors can avoid contact with difficult patients
- Patients may feel rejected by doctor and fail to attend
- Patients may feel worse after counselling
- Financial costs

DTB in July 2000

Limited evidence that in the short-term brief counselling
- Leads to better psychological symptom control
- Increases patient satisfaction
- Decreases mental health referrals
- Seems to work best in response to specific needs (e.g. bereavement, psycho-sexual, relationships, family breakdown)
- Reduces prescribing of psychotropic drugs

However
- Studies are small and would not stand up well to rigorous appraisal
- GPs should employ only those counsellors who are registered with the British Association of Counsellors
- Conclusion once again was 'more data needed'

CHAPTER 5: THE ELDERLY

THE 'GREY ARMY'

The unexpected improvements in average life expectancy in the 20th century have thrust ageing to the forefront of attention. More old people are alive today than at any time in history.

People over 60 currently constitute 20% of the UK population and will constitute 33% by 2030. The numbers of people with chronic diseases and disabilities are also projected to increase 2–3 fold. Increasing life expectancy is hailed by some as one of the greatest achievements of the 20th century, a more common reaction is a doom-laden prediction of health and social budgets being drained by caring for dependent old people. Some have argued that directing resources away from old people can be justified. Sensible debate has been hampered by hysterical media coverage.

The Elderly

IMPLICATIONS FOR HEALTH CARE

- Evidence exists that the functional health of the population is improving
- Proportion of men and women at any age who require help with four activities of daily living halved between 1976 and 1991
- If trends continue it could greatly reduce the numbers of people needing health care
- Conversely the numbers of people with hip fracture has increased in the last decade
- Importance of trying to reduce hip fractures was emphasised in a recent paper from Australia when 80% of the elderly women said that they would rather die than suffer a bad hip fracture and be admitted to a nursing home *(BMJ 2000;320:341–6)*
- Evidence exists that modifiable environmental and lifestyle factors are important determinants of disease in old age
- It is therefore a priority to understand the causes and prevention of chronic disease, disability and maintaining good health in an ageing society
- May need to change the emphasis of medical education
- Increasing sub-specialisation in medicine produces doctors who are unable to deal with the multiple pathology found in most elderly people
- This gives strength to the position of GPs as generalists

The Elderly

IMPLICATIONS FOR SOCIETY

- Decline of the family unit means that fewer elderly people cared for by their relatives
- In the NHS Plan the Government has agreed that nursing care should be provided free of charge
- Problem of ageism in clinical medicine and in health policy
- Less likely to get potentially life saving/enhancing investigation and treatment as patients get older
- Ageism also occurs in prevention of heart disease although evidence suggests most likely to benefit
- Older patients usually excluded from large RCTs and therefore significantly under represented in the evidence base used to determine clinical effectiveness
- Clinical guidelines when developed should take into account the elderly as an equal treatment group with their own priorities
- The elderly have as much right to health promotion and disease prevention as younger patients
- Older people should be informed of the choices and standards of care offered
- Possible questions on dementia and related topics are bountiful especially in terms of ethics, duty of care etc.
- Remember to mention and give examples if required of patient consent, end of life decisions and advance directives (see page 195).

Q. Views on withdrawal of treatment/feeding – is it ethical to withdraw?
Q. Dealing with relatives and request by third parties for sedation.

National Service Framework (NSF) for Older People

The original document is over 100 pages long, as such the salient points have been summarised with respect to General Practice. This NSF is a 10 year strategy to ensure fair, high quality, integrated health and social care services for older people. It is designed to support independence and promote good health. Aims to promote and engender that older people and their carers are always treated with respect, dignity and fairness. The National Director for Older People, Professor Ian Philp, will lead NSF implementation.

The Elderly

The four themes in this NSF are:
1. Respecting the individual
2. Intermediate care
3. Providing evidence-based specialist care
4. Promoting an active, healthy life

Prior to this NSF some action has already taken place through other initiatives:

Improving standards of care
*   In rest/nursing homes, through the new National Care Standards Commission and through the *Better Care, Higher Standards Charters*

Extending access to services
*   Free NHS sight tests for those aged 60 and over
*   Improved access to cataract services
*   Extension of breast screening to women aged up to 70
*   Carers' access to services in their own right has been ensured through the *Carers and Disabled Children Act 2000*
*   *Care Direct* (Government pilot), a one-stop shop gateway to information about social care, health, housing and social security benefits, which will complement *NHS Direct*
*   DoH issued *Fair Access to Care Services* guidance to councils in Spring 2001 setting out how they should develop fair and consistent eligibility criteria for adult social care services

Developing services which support independence
*   *Promoting Independence Grant* supports councils to help more people to retain their independence for longer.
*   *Supporting People* is a new initiative to help vulnerable people live independently in the community by providing a wide range of housing support services

Helping older people to stay healthy
*   Free influenza immunisation for everyone aged 65 and over
*   Improve oral health in older people and increase access to dentistry through *Modernising NHS Dentistry*
*   Routine breast cancer screening is being extended to women up to the age of 70
*   *Keep Warm, Keep Well* campaigns to prevent deaths in winter and increased Winter Fuel Payments of £200

The Elderly

Ensuring fairer funding
- End the anomaly that people in nursing homes may have to pay for their nursing care, it will be provided on the same basis as other NHS services, free at the point of use
- 3 months property disregard and by raising the capital limits when councils may step in with financial support
- Deferred payment scheme, to be introduced from October 2001, will give people more choice in how they pay for residential accommodation
- Aim to give people a valuable breathing space between entering a care home and selling their home, if that is their wish

Developing more effective links between health and social services
- The Health Act 1999 allowed partnership between Health Authorities and councils to improve services at the interface of health and social care
- Local Strategic Partnerships (LSPs) will be established across the country from April 2001
  - Committed to improving the quality of life
  - Refocusing of mainstream services and resources
  - LSPs will bring together the public, private, voluntary and community sectors and service users to provide a single overarching local framework that will allow NSFs to be implemented

The NSF itself had eight standards, each accompanied with details of arrangements that would allow it to be implemented. (As you go through the standards note which have any additional funding in order to aid implementation.)

STANDARD 1: ROOTING OUT AGE DISCRIMINATION

NHS services will be provided, regardless of age, on the basis of clinical need alone. Social care services will not use age in their eligibility criteria or policies, to restrict access to available services.

- Negative staff attitudes also impact on the quality of care
- Palliative care services have not been available to older people in some areas
- This may be related to the fact that palliative care services have been concentrated on those with cancer rather than terminal stages of a chronic disorder
- Elderly people from black and minority ethnic groups can be

The Elderly

disadvantaged and are likely to suffer more discrimination in accessing services
- Concerns have been raised about resuscitation policies with older people more likely to be denied cardiopulmonary resuscitation (CPR) on the grounds of age alone; Guidelines from the BMA, RCN and Resuscitation Council suggest regular audits of local CPR policies in order to prevent age related discrimination
- Denying access to services on the basis of age alone is not acceptable
- Decisions should be made on the basis of health needs and ability to benefit, rather than age
- National guidance will be developed by May 2001 to assist with the audits of age-related policies
- Age discrimination may not always be explicit

STANDARD 2: PERSON-CENTRED CARE

NHS and social care services treat older people as individuals and enable them to make choices about their own care. This can be achieved through the single assessment process, integrated commissioning arrangements and integrated provision of services, including community equipment and continence services.

The plan focused on key areas of improvement, where need was identified, they are summarized below.

Personal and professional behaviour
- Staff should be polite and courteous at all times (e.g. using the older person's preferred form of address and relating to them as a competent adult)
- Procedures are in place to identify and if possible meet, any particular needs and preferences relating to gender, personal appearance, communication, diet, race or culture and religious/spiritual beliefs
- Personal hygiene needs are met with sensitivity, intimate interventions carried out in privacy
- Patients allowed to wear their own clothes in hospital and able to have personal effects at their bedside (space/safety permitting)

Dignity in end-of-life care
- Control of painful and distressing symptoms
- Rehabilitation and support as health declines

The Elderly

- Social care to maintain access to safe and accessible living environments, practical help, income maintenance, social networks and information
- Spiritual care – availability of pastoral or spiritual carers reflecting the faiths of the local population
- Provide evidence-based complementary therapies
- Psychological care to anticipate, recognise and treat any psychological distress of the patient or carer
- Bereavement support and counselling

The single assessment process
- Proposed by The NHS Plan
- To be introduced April 2002, for health and social care for older people
- Covers health and social care for older people
- Standardised assessment process is in place across all areas and agencies
- Raised standards of assessment
- Designed to identify all of their needs
- Less duplication and worry for the patient
- Can be carried out by one front-line professional
- If other professionals need to be involved this will be arranged to provide a seamless service
- Assessment scales and tools are validated

Integrated community equipment services
- Audit Commission estimated that nearly 1 million people need equipment to help them live independently
- Demand for disability equipment is increasing due to ageing population and user expectation
- The NHS Plan set out an intention to achieve single, integrated community equipment services by 2004 and to increase by 50% the number of people able to benefit; comes with increased funding

Integrated continence services
- Primary and community staff involved in the identification and initial assessment and care
- Specialist services to provide expert advice when condition does not respond to initial treatment
- Availability and provision of continence aids/equipment and access to bathing/laundry services

The Elderly

STANDARD 3: INTERMEDIATE CARE

Older people will have access to a new range of intermediate care services at home or in designated care settings, to promote their independence by providing enhanced services from the NHS and councils to prevent unnecessary hospital admission and effective rehabilitation services to enable early discharge from hospital and to prevent premature or unnecessary admission to long-term residential care.

- A new layer of care, between primary care and specialist services
- To prevent unnecessary hospital admission, support early discharge and reduce or delay long-term residential care
- To improve physical functioning, build confidence, re-equip with the skills they need to live safely and independently at home
- Rehabilitation reduces re-admittance to hospitals and long terms in residential care
- Rehabilitation improves survival rates and physical and cognitive functioning
- 63% of older people permanently enter nursing home care, 43% of those entering residential care homes come direct from hospital
- Older people will be the main but not exclusive beneficiaries of these services
- Should involve rapid assessment, diagnosis and immediate treatment followed by appropriate referral
- Will include counselling, intensive support at home for a short period, community nursing and therapy services ('hospital at home')
- Well-managed intermediate care can improve recovery rates, increase patient satisfaction and reduce impact on the primary care team
- Strongest evidence is for stroke rehabilitation and geriatric/orthopaedic rehabilitation (more patients being discharged home compared with conventional care)

STANDARD 4: GENERAL HOSPITAL CARE

Older people's care in hospital is delivered through appropriate specialist care and by hospital staff who have the right set of skills to meet their needs.

Emergency response
- Older people should be transferred from A&E as soon as possible

The Elderly

- The NHS Plan commitment is that no patient should stay longer than 4 hours in A&E (by 2004)

Early assessment
- Should identify the further care the older person requires
- Will include investigation, observation and multidisciplinary assessment
- Input from geriatricians, specialists in stroke, falls and mental health or other disciplines including specialist nurses, therapists, pharmacists and social workers, may be required
- Clinical Leaders (Modern Matrons) for Older People to oversee care

Appropriate surroundings
- Separate room always available for private discussions and to make personal telephone calls
- Building design or re-design should take the need for privacy into account
- More four-bedded bays
- Single rooms for the most vulnerable
- Space provided for therapy equipment, or a small gym, comfortable day rooms and specially adapted kitchens
- 95% of NHS accommodation will be single sex by 2002

STANDARD 5: STROKE

The NHS will take action to prevent strokes, working in partnership with other agencies where appropriate. People who are thought to have had a stroke have access to diagnostic services, are treated appropriately by a specialist stroke service, and subsequently, with their carers, participate in a multidisciplinary programme of secondary prevention and rehabilitation.

- Each year 110,000 people in England and Wales have their first stroke (30,000 have further strokes); biggest cause of severe disability and the third most common cause of death in the UK
- 30% of patients die in the first month after a stroke
- After a year, 65% of surviving stroke patients can live independently, 35% are significantly disabled
- Around 5% are admitted to long-term residential care
- Risk increases with age but young people affected too
- 10,000 people under 55 years and 1,000 people under 30 years have a stroke each year

The Elderly

- African-Caribbean and South Asian men are about 40% and 70% more likely to have a stroke
- Socio-economic group V have a 60% higher chance of having a stroke than group I
- Mortality rates from stroke are 50% higher in socio-economic group V than in group I
- Strong evidence that people who have a stroke are more likely both to survive and to recover more function if admitted promptly to a hospital based stroke unit
- Apparently the NSF states this can be achieved at no overall additional cost to health and social care!
- By April 2002 every DGH which cares for people with stroke will have plans to introduce a specialised stroke service
- By April 2003 RCP guidelines for stroke care will be in place and audited
- By April 2004 PCG/Ts will have ensured that:
  - Every GP is using protocols agreed with local specialist services
  - Identifying and treating patients identified as being at risk
  - Rapid referral and management of those with TIA – guidelines in place

Population approaches to preventing stroke
- Similar to those for coronary heart disease – increasing levels of physical activity, encouraging healthy eating, supporting smoking cessation and identifying and managing high blood pressure

Preventing strokes in individuals at greater risk

Main risk factors
Cardiovascular disease
hypertension, atrial fibrillation, CHD previous stroke or TIA, peripheral vascular disease, carotid stenosis
Metabolic
diabetes, hyperlipidaemia and obesity
Lifestyle
alcohol misuse, poor diet, low level of physical activity and smoking

- Risk of stroke for people with hypertension can be reduced by 37% through treatment
- Atrial fibrillation increases the risk of having a stroke by 3–7 times
- 13% of people who have had a stroke are in atrial fibrillation
- In the younger population risk factors include sickle cell disease,

The Elderly

congenital heart disease, abnormalities of blood clotting and arterio-venous malformations of the brain.

Long-term support
Can continue over a long time and until maximum recovery has been achieved.

Some will need ongoing support and have access to a stroke care co-ordinator who can provide advice, arrange reassessment, co-ordinate long-term support or arrange for specialist care.

Any patient reporting a significant disability at six months should be re-assessed and offered further targeted rehabilitation, if this can help recover further function.

STANDARD 6: FALLS

The NHS, working in partnership with councils, takes action to prevent falls and reduce resultant fractures or other injuries in their populations of older people. Older people who have fallen receive effective treatment and rehabilitation and, with their carers, receive advice on prevention, through a specialised falls service.

- Falls are the leading cause of mortality due to injury in older people aged over 75 in the UK
- 14,000 people a year die in the UK as a result of an osteoporotic hip fracture
- Osteoporotic fractures occur most commonly in the hip, spine and wrist
- One third of women and one twelfth of men over 50 are affected by osteoporosis
- 50% of women have an osteoporotic fracture by the time they reach the age of 70
- Consequences for an individual of falling or of not being able to get up after a fall can include:
  - Psychological problems, for example a fear of falling and loss of confidence
  - Loss of mobility leading to social isolation and depression
  - Increase in dependency and disability
  - Hypothermia
  - Pressure-related injury
  - Infection

The Elderly

- After an osteoporotic fracture, 50% can no longer live independently
- Falls are a common symptom of previously unidentified health problems

Prevention
- Older people who have fallen are at risk of falling again
- A specialist falls services should be established for older people

Population approach to falls prevention
- Reduce incidence and impact of falls through encouraging appropriate weight-bearing and strength enhancing physical activity, promoting healthy eating and reducing smoking
- Community strategy to prevent falls should also include:
  - Ensuring that pavements are kept clear and in good repair
  - Adequate street lighting
  - Providing information, such as '*Avoiding Slips, Trips and Broken Hips*' by the Department of Trade and Industry (Dti)
  - Making property safer

 USEFUL WEBSITE

www.preventinghomefalls.gov.uk

Preventing falls in individuals
- Depends on identifying those most at risk
- Many who fall do not seek medical help but may be identified through risk factors
- Interventions should target both multiple risk factors for individuals (intrinsic risk factors) and environmental hazards to be successful

Intrinsic risk factors include
- Balance, gait or mobility problems including those due to degenerative joint disease and motor disorders such as stroke and Parkinson's disease
- Taking four or more medications, in particular centrally sedating or blood pressure lowering drugs
- Visual impairment
- Impaired cognition or depression
- Postural hypotension

The Elderly

Risk factors in the home environment include
- Poor lighting, particularly on stairs
- Steep stairs
- Loose carpets or rugs
- Slippery floors
- Badly fitting footwear or clothing
- Lack of safety equipment such as grab rails
- Inaccessible lights or windows

Assessment of risk of osteoporosis

Risk factors for osteoporosis include
- Previous fragility fracture (e.g. wrists)
- Prolonged corticosteroid therapy
- Hysterectomy, premature menopause or history of amenorrhoea (not treated to reduce risk of osteoporosis)
- Risk factors such as liver or thyroid disease, malabsorption, alcoholism, rheumatoid arthritis and male hypogonadism
- Family history of osteoporosis (including maternal hip fracture)
- Low body mass <19 kg/m^2
- Smoking

Treating osteoporosis
- When patients are identified as being at high-risk bone mineral density measurement should be carried out in line with the RCP Clinical Guidelines
- All patients get lifestyle advice on nutrition (calcium and vitamin D), regular weight bearing exercise, stopping smoking and avoiding alcohol
- Drug interventions: HRT, selective oestrogen receptor modulators (SERMS) and bisphosphonates will be most cost-effective when prescribed in high risk older people
- Frail or housebound people with previous fragility fractures may benefit from supplements of calcium and vitamin D to help prevent hip fracture

STANDARD 7: MENTAL HEALTH IN OLDER PEOPLE

Older people who have mental health problems have access to integrated mental health services, provided by the NHS and councils to ensure effective diagnosis, treatment and support, for them and for their carers.

The Elderly

- Cost of care for Alzheimer's Disease (AD) in 1993 was estimated at over £1 billion
- Considerable variation across the country exists in mental health services for older people
- Under-detection of mental illness in older people is widespread
- Depression in people aged 65 and over is especially under-diagnosed
- Mental and physical problems interact in older people making diagnosis and management difficult
- Older people from black and minority ethnic communities need accessible and appropriate mental health services
- Assessments may be culturally biased
- Information about services may not be effective if this relies on translated leaflets or posters rather than more appropriate mechanisms
- There may be distrust of agencies by some black and minority ethnic communities
- Older people with learning disabilities may have difficulty obtaining appropriate mental health care
- Family or paid carers of disabled elderly may not be alert to their mental health needs

Promoting mental health
- Standard 8 sets out the interventions at population level to promote good mental health
- Additional interventions which will promote mental health include tackling social isolation, providing bereavement support and suicide prevention
- Key elements of suicide prevention will include health maintenance and promotion, treatment of depression in primary care and screening for suicidal ideation coupled with prevention
- Older people in residential care and nursing homes should be able to participate in a range of stimulating group or one to one activities

Depression
- 10–15% of the population aged 65 and over will have depression
- More severe states of depression are less common, affecting about 3–5% of older people
- Depression severely affects the quality of life and may adversely affect physical health

The Elderly

- Depression may be triggered by a variety of factors such as bereavement and loss, life changes such as unemployment, retirement and social isolation
- Older people can also become depressed because of increasing illness or frailty, or following a stroke or a fall
- Early recognition can reduce distressing symptoms and prevent physical illness, adverse effects upon social relationships, self-neglect and self-harm or suicide

Dementia

Dementia is a clinical syndrome characterised by a widespread loss of mental function, with the following features:
- Memory loss
- Language impairment (having difficulty finding words especially names and nouns)
- Disorientation (not knowing the time or place)
- Change in personality (becoming more irritable, anxious or withdrawn; loss of skills and impaired judgement)
- Self neglect
- Behaviour that is out of character (for example, sexual disinhibition or aggression)

Dementia has a number of causes, the most common of which are:
- AD – responsible for 60% of dementia cases, characterised by memory loss and difficulties with language becoming more severe over several years
- Vascular dementia – this is the consequence of strokes and/or insufficient blood flow to the brain and causes up to 20% of cases of dementia; signs depend on area of brain involved
- AD and vascular dementia can co-exist
- Dementia with Lewy bodies – this causes up to 15% of dementia cases and is characterised by symptoms similar to Parkinson's Disease as well as hallucinations
- Approximately 600,000 people in the UK have dementia (5% of the total population aged 65 and over, rising to 20% over the age of 80)
- 17,000 people with dementia are in younger age groups
- 154,000 live alone with dementia
- By 2026 there will be 840,000 people with dementia in the UK, rising to 1.2 million by 2050
- People diagnosed should be assessed under the single assessment process

The Elderly

STANDARD 8: THE PROMOTION OF HEALTH AND ACTIVE LIFE IN OLDER AGE

The health and well-being of older people is promoted through a co-ordinated programme of action led by the NHS with support from councils.

- NHS and local partners should re-focus on helping older people to continue to live healthy and fulfilling lives
- Growing body of evidence to suggest modification of risk factors late in life can have health benefits; longer life, increased/maintained levels of functional ability, disease prevention and an improved sense of well-being
- Integrated strategies for older people aimed at promoting good health and quality of life and to prevent or delay frailty and disability can have significant benefits for the individual and society

Action can be taken by the NHS and councils to:
- Prevent or delay the onset of ill health and disability
- Reduce the impact of illness and disability on health and well-being
- Identify barriers to healthy living (for example cultural appropriateness of services)
- Working with council services such as leisure and lifelong learning
- Health promotion activity should take account of differences in lifestyle and the impact of cultural/religious beliefs, for example it would not be appropriate to advise a strict Muslim woman to take up a certain form of exercise which would mean that she would have to wear scant clothes for exercise or be in the same room as men.

PAPERS:

A series of four articles appeared in the BMJ in March and April 2001. They focused on the care of elderly, the basis being extensive literature reviews undertaken to inform the development of the National Service Framework (NSF) for NHS care of older people in England. Some of the issues mentioned are covered in the NSF. Salient points are listed overleaf along with any general issues that may arise.

The Elderly

▨ *Care of older people – Maintaining the dignity and autonomy of older people in the healthcare setting.*
(BMJ 2001;322:668)

- It appeared that it is not just the lack of autonomy of elderly people within the healthcare service but a somewhat unsettling lack of respect for their dignity
- Autonomy and dignity although related are differing concepts
- Dignity referring to an individual maintaining self respect and being valued by others
- Autonomy refers to individual control of decision making and other activities
- Both the dignity and the autonomy of older people are often undermined in healthcare settings
- Negative interactions between staff and patients, a lack of regard for patients' privacy and a general insensitivity to the needs and desires of an older population all effect their 'dignity'
- 'Autonomy is threatened when patients (and their carers) are not given adequate information or the opportunity to understand fully their diagnosis and to make informed choices about their care'
- Qualitative data cited in the article suggests that attitudes of staff greatly affect both the quality of treatment of older people and the regard given to maintaining their dignity and autonomy
- Older people are becoming disempowered in healthcare settings
- Not just a problem in the UK but internationally
- Pessimistic viewpoints of healthcare professionals translate into a loss of dignity, identity and decision-making power for seniors
- Ageism, it appears, is as much of a problem within the NHS as it is within the population as a whole
- 'Tackling negative attitudes through exposure and education can help to preserve older patients' dignity and autonomy'
- 'Giving older people and their carers adequate information for them to make informed choices about care further increases autonomy'

The ironic realization is that the issues facing our profession in caring for the elderly are the same as those the western world so readily counts as one of its merits, namely Autonomy, Dignity and Equality.

From articles such as those listed above and guidelines such as the NSF it is envisaged we can go someway in closing the apparent gap that exists between the young and the old.

The Elderly

 Promoting health and function in an ageing population.
(BMJ 2001;322:728)

The second article was written by an Australian academic in *'Ageing Studies'*. Through a review of literature he looked at the evidence of the effectiveness of strategies for promoting health and function, particularly the benefits of exercise in old age.

- The prevalence of disability in older people is declining
- In order to maintain health and function in the elderly, the social, mental, economic and environmental determinants of health in old age must be taken into account
- The health benefits of exercise may often relate to psychosocial as well as direct health gains
- Most health benefits can be gained from regular physical activity of moderate intensity
- Health and well-being at older ages is modifiable
- Promoting health and fitness throughout life could make substantial gains
- The World Health Organisation (WHO) has argued for a proactive and positive approach to dealing with the risk of chronic disease in old age
- WHO proposed a 'life course' approach for dealing with the health issues associated with ageing and recommended implementing programmes that are oriented towards positive interventions in earlier life

The third article looked at the quality of mental health services for the elderly.

 Care of Older People – Mental Health Problems
(BMJ 2001;322:789)

The paper outlined the current evidence of benefit in four areas: services currently available; interventions that have been shown to be effective; rating scales that should be recommended to clinicians for detecting common mental health problems; and the needs of carers.

- Guidelines and standardised screening instruments improve recognition
- Carer interventions in people with dementia have been shown to be effective in RCTs
- Depression is the commonest mental health disorder and psychological therapies are underused

The Elderly

- Memory clinics improve significantly the quality of life in carers of people with dementia because of the treatment and advice they offer
- A randomised controlled trial of a psychiatric liaison intervention for medical inpatients aged over 75, showed that those in the intervention group had improved physical function, fewer readmissions to hospital or nursing home and a shorter length of stay
- A similar intervention was shown to be effective in frail, older people living at home

 Falls in late life and their consequences
(BMJ 2001;322:855)

The last in this series of articles looked at falls in the elderly. The salient points were covered in the NSF but it would be a relatively easy read if you wanted more detail.

The Elderly

DEMENTIA

Incidence of 1.6 and a prevalence of 3.6 patients per year.

 North of England Evidence-Based Guidelines
(BMJ 1998;317:802)
- Subjective complaints of memory loss are not a good indicator of dementia
- GPs should use formal cognitive testing to enhance their judgement (short MMTS)
- Routine blood and urine screening tests should be done
- Exclude diagnosis of Lewy body dementia (fluctuations with paranoid delusions, auditory and visual hallucinations, clouding of consciousness and depression) as greatly increased morbidity and mortality associated with use of neuroleptic drugs
- Look for depression, as it is common and a trial of anti-depressants may be helpful
- Underlying causes (physical, social, environmental) for any sudden behavioural change should be sought
- Falls and hip fracture are very common and active prevention is necessary
- Remember the carer

Treatment of Alzheimer's disease (AD)
- Increasing evidence that anticholinesterase inhibitors have a real, if modest, benefit in AD
- Review in Cochrane in 1998 showed significant improvements in 'cognitive decline scores' and 'clinical global impression' for treatment of 12–24 weeks in mild to moderate AD, but NO improvement in quality of life scores
- Recently Rivastigmine has been assessed in an international RCT *(BMJ 1999;318:633)*. Patients with mild to moderate AD over 6 months of treatment showed:
  - increased cognitive scores
  - improved carer rated quality of life
  - increased function and ADL
  - improved global clinical assessment
- First study to show improvement in ADL, quality of life and cognitive scores

However, benefits are modest, costs high and all the patients receive a very detailed assessment which in itself may be beneficial.

NICE Guideline – on the use of Donepezil, Rivastigmine and Galantamine for the treatment of AD.
(Jan 2001)
- Available on the NHS as part of the management for mild and moderate AD
- For patients with MMSE score of >12/30
- Only specialists should initiate treatment
- Agreed shared-care protocol with GPs
- Reviewed at 2 to 4 months
- Continue only if MMSE >12

Evidence
NICE performed a systematic review of 5 RCTs for donepezil, 5 for rivastigmine and 3 for galantamine. Also used unpublished studies from drug companies. All three drugs show statistically significant improvement in cognitive function compared with placebo.

Typical average improvements of 1 to 2 points in MMSE (out of 30 points) over 6 months are usual compared with placebo. Compared with an average decline of some 4 or 5 points per year in placebo-treated patients within trials. RCT evidence of improvement in quality of life measures is less positive. There is no measure of quality of life for use in patients with dementia that has proved universally satisfactory. Evidence that quality of life has been improved by any of these drugs has therefore been mixed. Carers report functional benefits and improvement in behavioural symptoms, such as agitation and aggression, as well as in motivation, concentration, control and independence. Placebo effects are quite large, with as many as 30% improving on baseline outcome scores at the next assessment.

Clinical Evidence 2000
Beneficial: Donepezil
Likely to be beneficial: Rivastigmine, Selegiline (one systematic review) and Gingko

DTB February 2000
Looked at new evidence looking at aspirin, anti-inflammatory drugs and free radical scavengers and concluded that they 'remain unconvinced' of its value.

Gingko biloba
Extracts of Gingko biloba (Bandolier 18) have a modest effect. Over one

year the NNT is 7 for an improved cognitive decline score and for the patients family to notice a difference. The dose is 40 mg tds.

PAPERS:

 Statins can help prevent dementia
(*Scott. BMJ 18 November 2000.*)

Looked at two new studies showing statins may also reduce the risk of Alzheimer's disease and other dementias.
- First study used data from 368 medical practices in the UK, researchers compared data from 284 patients with Alzheimer's disease and other dementias with 1080 controls without dementia
- People taking statins were about 70% less likely to have dementia than people who had not been diagnosed with high lipid concentrations or who were taking other lipid-lowering drugs (*Lancet 2000;356:1627*)
- Statins seem to do more than just lower cholesterol concentrations since patients taking other lipid-lowering drugs had no significant decrease in dementia when compared with patients without high cholesterol

Epidemiological study in Archives of Neurology (October 2000) showed:
- People on statins had a lower risk of developing Alzheimer's disease
- Proposed that the effect is because statins raise concentrations of endothelial nitric oxide synthase, allowing the microvasculature flexibility and therefore increased blood flow

Scientists still do not know which mechanism is responsible for this outcome. Because of its design the latest study cannot provide a conclusive answer.

Wealthier, educated people, who tend to be at lower risk of dementia, may be more likely to take cholesterol-lowering drugs. RCT needed where people randomly assigned to take cholesterol lowering drugs or placebo and then followed over time to see who develops dementia.

 A healthy old age: realistic or futile goal?
(*McMurdo. BMJ 2000;321:1149–51*)
This interesting article looked at beliefs and myths regarding old age. It focused on exercise and healthy living.

The Elderly

- Although older people have poorer health than younger people, ageing does not cause disease
- Older people with better health habits live healthier for longer
- Regular physical activity in old age can 'rejuvenate' physical capacity by 10–15 years
- Regular moderate intensity activity for 30 minutes on most days of the week benefits health
- Activity need not be continuous and may be accumulated in short bouts
- Physical activity levels are related to income and inversely related to age
- Older people who have long been sedentary should start slowly, beginning with a few minutes a day and build up gradually
- If an activity is not provoking symptoms it is very unlikely to be doing harm
- For most older people the benefits of activity outweigh the risks
- Clinicians should be physically active, to benefit their own health and to add credibility to their advice!

CHAPTER 6: OBSTETRICS & GYNAECOLOGY

COMBINED ORAL CONTRACEPTIVE PILL

The combined oral contraceptive pill (COCP) has been one of the most extensively researched medicines and is still providing many areas of controversy and discussion. The Pill continues to be one of the most worried and talked about drugs, regularly making newspaper headlines. Consequently, women's fears persist out of all proportion to actual risk, and in most cases women are unaware of the Pill's substantial non-contraceptive health benefits. In addition, the medical professionals knowledge of the pill's advantages and disadvantages is still very varied. Two large cohort studies followed a total of over 70,000 women and had very reassuring results with the same mortality rates for users and non-users.

What is the risk of deep vein thrombosis to women taking the combined oral contraceptive?
The largest area of controversy is the increased risk of deep vein thrombosis (DVT) with third generation pills.

In October 1995 the Committee on Safety of Medicines warned that COCP containing desogestrel or gestodene carried a small increased risk of DVT compared with other preparations so should not be used as first-line treatment. Subsequent studies have actually shown no difference in risk of thromboembolism between different pill preparations.

However, two different studies in the BMJ have used the same data and reported opposite conclusions regarding the risk of DVT in third generation oral contraceptives! *(BMJ 2000;321:477–9, 1190–5)*. However, the superior design and analysis of the more recent study *(BMJ 2000;321:1190–5)* mean that it could be the most important paper yet published on this vexed subject. It also provides vital evidence on several controversial matters, including the increased risk in first time users of oral contraceptives and the role of risk factors such as obesity and smoking. It showed that women with a BMI of at least 35 have a four-fold increased risk of DVT by taking all types of combined oral contraceptives.

Obstetrics & Gynaecology

The quoted risks of DVT are as follows:

Non-users	5 :100 000
2nd generation pill	15 :100 000
3rd generation pill	30 :100 000
Pregnancy	60 :100 000

The Department of Health actually announced in 1999 an end to the 1995 restrictions on prescribing 3rd generation oral contraceptive pills. The absolute risk of venous thromboembolism in women taking either 2nd or 3rd generation combined oral contraceptives remains very small and still well below the risk associated with pregnancy. Provided that the women are informed of and accept the relative risks of thromboembolism, the choice of oral contraceptive is for the woman and the prescriber to decide jointly in the light of her individual medical history and any contraindications.

Is there an increased risk of myocardial infarction?
A recent large community based case-control study found no association between the use of the combined oral contraceptive and myocardial infarction, and no difference of risk between 2nd and 3rd generation pills *(BMJ 1999;318:1579-84)*. The risk of myocardial infarction in women taking the combined oral contraceptive seems to increase only in association with additional risk factors (e.g. smoking, diabetes, obesity, hypertension). The combined oral contraceptive pill is contraindicated in women with severe or multiple risk factors for ischaemic heart disease.

Is there an increased risk of ischaemic stroke?
In women who do not smoke and do not have hypertension, the risk of ischaemic stroke is 1.5 times higher than in non-users. However, the risk rises to threefold in women with hypertension taking the combined oral contraceptive.

Is there an increased risk of haemorrhagic stroke?
There is no increased risk in women under the age of 35 years who are non-smokers and normotensive. One study has shown that women over 35 years have a double risk of haemorrhagic stroke compared with non-users. Women who smoke and take the pill are three times more likely to have a haemorrhagic stroke, and hypertensive women have a 10–15 times increased risk.

Does taking the combined oral contraceptive pill lead to hypertension?

Obstetrics & Gynaecology

There is a lack of data on the effects of the low dose combined oral contraceptive on blood pressure. If a woman develops pill-induced hypertension she should consider an alternative method of contraception. The pill should not be used and also be stopped in patients with a sustained blood pressure above 160/95 mmHg.

Is the combined oral contraceptive pill contraindicated in women with migraine?

The incidence of ischaemic (not haemorrhagic) stroke is increased in women with migraine, particularly if they are also taking the combined oral contraceptive pill *(BMJ 1999;318:13–18)*. The combined oral contraceptive pill is contraindicated in patients who have migraines with focal aura (migraine with focal symptoms) or classical migraine and those patients who have severe migraines lasting over 72 hours despite treatment.

Are there benefits from taking the combined oral contraceptive pill?

It is important to remember that the Pill has numerous advantages. These include:

- Excellent efficacy and acceptability
- Beneficial effects on menstrual disorders
- Suppression of benign breast disease
- Protection against endometrial and ovarian cancer
- Protection against pelvic inflammatory disease.

Any adverse effects from taking the oral contraceptive pill are reversed after 10 years cessation of the pill.

SUMMARY POINTS FOR COMBINED ORAL CONTRACEPTION

- ❖ Very safe and effective contraception
- ❖ Conflicting evidence still exists regarding thrombotic risk
- ❖ Absolute risk of DVT very small with 3rd generation pill
- ❖ Always consider patient's risk factors for CHD

EMERGENCY CONTRACEPTION

Emergency contraception (also called postcoital contraception) is a safe and highly effective way of preventing an accidental pregnancy; it is not suitable if used as a regular method of birth control.

Levonelle-2 has recently been launched as a progesterone-only emergency contraception pill. It prevents pregnancy by suppressing ovulation, impairing fallopian transport of the egg and sperm (so preventing fertilisation) and also prevents implantation of any fertilised egg.

Levonelle-2 appears to be very safe and there are no contraindications for its use. It is more effective than PC4, as illustrated in the graph below. The percentage of pregnancies prevented is 95% compared with 77% with PC4 within 24 hours and 85% compared with 77% within 72 hours. This increased efficacy if taken early illustrates that ease of access to the drug is crucial for its effectiveness. It has been associated with a much lower incidence of side-effects (especially vomiting).

Graph to illustrate the efficacy of Levonelle-2 compared with PC4

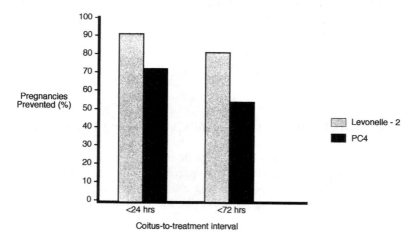

Levonelle-2 has recently been available from designated pharmacists in Manchester as part of a six month pilot study. 3500 women used the service, 24% were teenagers and 18% live outside the area, reflecting the high demand for this service. Pharmacists were given a £10 fee for each script. The trial was actually extended due to its popularity.

Obstetrics & Gynaecology

A medicine must have prescription-only status, if there would be a danger to health if the substance were used without medical supervision; the product might be used incorrectly, so endangering health; and the active ingredient, or side-effects it may cause, require further investigation. The Committee on Safety of Medicines advised that Levonelle-2 does not meet these criteria and so could be safely supplied by a pharmacist without medical supervision. The UK Government has taken this advice and recently announced that Levonelle-2 is available at a cost of £20, to women over 16 years (from pharmacies) without a doctor's prescription from 1 January 2001.

What are the advantages of Levonelle-2 being available without prescription?
- Very safe medication (unlike paracetamol and brufen!)
- Very effective medication
- Increases ease of access
- Patients may prefer anonymity
- Leads to reduction in unwanted pregnancies
- Supported by RCOG and BMA
- May save money by reduction in termination rates

What are the disadvantages of Levonelle-2 being available over the counter?
- Does not address on-going contraception and sexually transmitted diseases
- Lost opportunity for counselling/education
- Patients will have to pay for it
- Disapproval from church/anti-abortion groups
- Need highly motivated pharmacists
- Not all pharmacies will have an area for discussing private issues
- Has recently been banned in Ireland

Should Levonelle-2 be available free over the counter?
It has been estimated that £1 spent on contraception actually saves £11 in subsequent NHS costs from an unplanned pregnancy so it could be argued that offering free over the counter emergency contraception releases money to spend on other services.

Lambert, Lewisham and Southwark Health Authority (which has one of the highest rates of teenage pregnancies and unwanted pregnancies in the UK) has recently allowed specially trained pharmacists to dispense Levonelle-2 free rather than charging £20.

Obstetrics & Gynaecology

Women still need to know how, when and where they can obtain emergency contraception free of charge through established NHS routes of supply. Emergency contraception still remains available free on prescription from General Practitioners, family planning clinics, youth clinics, walk-in centres, some genitourinary medicine and Accident and Emergency Departments.

PC4 is still available on prescription but it is recommended that Levonelle-2 should be prescribed as first-line emergency contraception due to its greater efficacy, despite the increased cost. The intra-uterine contraceptive device is still available as an alternative, is effective for up to five days after unprotected intercourse and is more effective than the hormonal methods.

SUMMARY POINTS FOR EMERGENCY CONTRACEPTION

- ❖ Levonelle-2 now obtainable without prescription
- ❖ Low incidence of side-effects
- ❖ Levonelle-2 should be given early to improve efficacy
- ❖ IUCD still more effective

Obstetrics & Gynaecology

TEENAGERS AND SEXUAL HEALTH

The UK has the highest teenage pregnancy rate in 15–19-year-olds in Western Europe. 35% of teenage pregnancies result in termination. Many teenagers are willing to run the risk of an unplanned pregnancy or catching a sexually transmitted disease because they fear that their parents will find out if they seek advice from their GP. Reduction in teenage pregnancy was one of the targets set for improvement during the 1990s in the Health of the Nation document; however, it was not met!

What are the problems?
Teenagers are often confused about where they can obtain contraceptive advice or treatment, whether it is legal and how to use the different contraceptive methods. In the UK approximately 50% of teenagers use contraception; this rate is much higher in USA and Denmark, which suggests a poorer access and knowledge rather than lower demand in the UK. In addition, 75% of teenage mothers admit to having unplanned pregnancies.

In 1995–7 the rate of increase of gonorrhoea among 15–19-year-olds was 45% and chlamydia was 53%. The results of a recent questionnaire survey sent to 1045 children aged 13–15 years showed that 54% believed they had to be over 16 years of age to access sexual health services *(BJGP 2000:50;550–4)*.

How should GPs be able to improve teenage heath?
The Fraser (previously Gillick) ruling clarifies the legal position of treating children under 16 years old without parental consent – see Fraser guidelines page 105.

It has been estimated in various surveys that at least a quarter of teenagers do not believe that their consultation will be confidential. Posters or leaflets in the surgery explaining the services available and the confidentiality issue may be useful. Patients must have easy access to emergency contraception. It can be useful to advertise local family planning and youth clinics as many patients prefer these clinics rather than seeing their own GP.

Doctors can and should advise on the effective use of contraception for their patients. There is evidence to show that practices with young female partners have significantly lower teenage pregnancy rates *(BMJ 2000:320;842–5)*.

103

Obstetrics & Gynaecology

Recent research on teenage pregnancies found that almost all the teenagers had visited a GP in the previous year and many of them had sought contraceptive advice during the consultation *(BMJ 2000: 321;486–9)*. More worryingly, teenagers who had terminations of their pregnancy were more likely to have received emergency contraception in the past.

It is clear therefore that GPs should follow up teenage patients to ensure they are using their contraception correctly. In addition, patients who receive emergency contraception should be started on regular contraception at the same time and then have clear follow-up arrangements.

Finally, there is currently a debate as to whether school nurses should be prescribing Levonelle-2 to girls under 16 years of age; in some areas this is already happening, much to the outrage of both parents and the media.

What is the recently launched multimedia campaign about teenage pregnancy?

A national multimedia campaign about teenage pregnancy has recently begun. This aims to give young people information about sex and contraception, including facts about the rising rates of sexually transmitted infections among teenagers and dispelling some 'urban myths' about sex. This is going to be achieved by using adverts in teen magazines, on local radio stations and other media.

Specifically, the campaign messages are:
- You can get free, confidential advice about contraception whatever your age
- If you are sexually active, use contraception, because of the risk of pregnancy and infections
- You choose when to have sex, no one else

Local sexual health services are expected to see a gradual increase in demand from teenagers as a result of this campaign. To ensure the services are accessible and trusted by teenagers, a best practice guidance has been developed by the Teenage Pregnancy Unit for the commissioning and provision of effective services for young people.

Contraception and young people under 16 years – the Fraser guidelines

A young person under 16 years may be given advice and may be prescribed contraception without parental consent if the following conditions are met:
- She understands the advice and is competent to consent to treatment
- You encourage her to inform her parent or guardian
- You believe she is likely to commence or continue sexual activity with or without contraception
- Her physical or mental health will suffer if she does not receive contraception advice or supplies
- Providing contraception is in her best interest

 USEFUL WEBSITE

www.teenagepregnancyunit.gov.uk – Teenage Pregnancy Unit's website

SUMMARY POINTS FOR TEENAGERS AND SEXUAL HEALTH

- UK has highest teenage pregnancy rate
- Most teenagers unaware of confidentiality
- Lower teenage pregnancy rates in practices with young female partners
- Many teenagers ignorant of contraception methods and their availability

Obstetrics & Gynaecology

CHLAMYDIA

Chlamydia is the commonest curable sexually transmitted disease in the industrialised world and is currently a huge problem in young, sexually active adults. Long-term consequences of chlamydia include increased pelvic pain; increased rate of ectopic pregnancies and increased infertility rates. This latter consequence often only becomes apparent during investigations at infertility clinics, as many patients are unaware of earlier infection with chlamydia.

Up to 70% of women and 50% men with infections are asymptomatic. The incidence has increased by 76% over the past five years; it has been estimated as affecting 1 in 12 women aged 16–24 years.

Why has the incidence of sexually transmitted infection, including chlamydia, increased by so much?
Some of the rise in incidence may be a reflection of improved detection. However, one of the major factors behind the recent rises in Western Europe is probably changing sexual behaviour. In addition, levels of awareness and fear of HIV and AIDS among people have declined, and the major fear is now of unintended pregnancy rather than a sexually transmitted infection *(BMJ 2001;322:1135–6)*.

How is chlamydia detected?
Chlamydia has traditionally been diagnosed by endocervical swabs, which have poor sensitivity. The detection of chlamydial infection in women is particularly difficult because 5–30% of infected women are infected only in the urethra, which is not detected by endocervical swab culture. The taking of endocervical or urethral swabs is an uncomfortable, time-consuming, and relatively expensive procedure that obviously requires a pelvic examination.

New tests are emerging which are more sensitive and preferable to previous tests. The Ligase Chain Reaction (LCR) on a sample of urine is more sensitive than endocervical swabs (90% vs 65% sensitivity).

Why not screen for chlamydia in UK?
There are currently successful screening programmes in USA and Sweden, which have resulted in a lower incidence of chlamydia. Screening is currently under consideration for <25 year olds, patients with symptoms, women seeking termination of pregnancy and women >25 years with a new partner.

However, there are many problems with introducing a successful screening programme in the UK. These are clearly documented in the report by the CMO's advisory group (see website). They include the psychological barriers of investigation, costs involved and methods of contact tracing. If contact tracing is not done effectively and efficiently then any screening programme would be wasted as treated patients would simply become reinfected and so negate any good done!

Before a national screening programme can be introduced there needs to be effective implementation of training and education for both staff and patients, which will have huge resource implications. Many women have never heard of chlamydia, let alone its consequences, so at present it would be very difficult to expect people to be screened for a disease they have never heard of.

Finally, screening for chlamydia is a very sensitive area as many women may feel 'targeted' by the introduction of this programme. It needs to be addressed and implemented properly for it to be successful in the UK. Ideally, for chlamydia screening to be successful there should be a multidisciplinary structured approach with comprehensive testing of agreed 'at risk' population with both effective and timely treatment of infected patients and effective tracing and treatment of sexual contacts.

 USEFUL WEBSITE

www.doh.gov.uk/chlamyd.htm – report of the Chief Medical Officer's expert advisory group on chlamydia

---

SUMMARY POINTS FOR CHLAMYDIA

- Chlamydia is most prevalent STD in UK
- Highest rates in females aged 16–24 years
- Most infections are asymptomatic
- Screening programme needs to be properly implemented
- Continued lack of public awareness of chlamydia

Obstetrics & Gynaecology

HORMONE REPLACEMENT THERAPY

This is always a topical subject and patients are often guided by inaccurate information they have read in the lay press so it is important to be able to reassure and educate them with reference to the recent literature. Much of the data regarding hormone replacement therapy (HRT) comes from observational trials, which results in bias, making studies difficult to interpret. Patients taking HRT are more likely to be healthier, well educated and compliant (quite different from most patients) which makes it very difficult to control bias in these studies. It has been estimated that currently one-third of perimenopausal and postmenopausal women in the UK are taking HRT.

Does HRT protect patients from coronary heart disease?
This is still the most controversial area. The HERS (Heart and Estrogen/Progestin Replacement) study was the first randomised prospective study of 2,763 postmenopausal women in America with established ischaemic heart disease. The data showed that in the first year the HRT treated group actually suffered more coronary events, but by three and four years there was a significantly lower rate of events *(JAMA 1998;280:605–13)*. Many critics of this study felt it was stopped too soon. From this study it is not possible to recommend HRT to women with established ischaemic heart disease at an older age.

However, various other studies have shown that patients taking HRT have lower levels of LDL-cholesterol and higher levels of HDL-cholesterol compared with patients taking a placebo. Further randomised controlled trials are underway in order to clarify the association of HRT and coronary heart disease.

Is HRT related to breast cancer?
The risk of breast cancer is very exaggerated in the lay press and this risk is usually the one that dissuades many women from taking HRT. Some studies have shown that women who take oestrogen after their menopause are more likely to develop breast cancer; others have established no link.

A meta-analysis of 51 epidemiological studies looked at 52,705 women with breast cancer compared to 108,411 without has shown that there is a small increased risk of breast cancer with long-term HRT *(Lancet 1997; 350:1047–59)*. The excess in numbers of cases depends upon the duration of HRT – 2:1000 on HRT for 5 years, 6:1000 for 10 years and

Obstetrics & Gynaecology

12:1000 for 15 years. This risk **only** applies to women over the age of 50 years, so women taking replacement HRT (e.g. post-oophorectomy) are not at any higher risk of breast cancer until they reach the age of 50 years.

Studies have shown that women using HRT after the menopause are actually more likely to have slow growing and highly curable types of breast cancers. An American study showed that women taking HRT had no difference in their risk of getting the fast growing, life-threatening tumours, ductal carcinoma in situ, invasive ductal or lobular cancer, which together constitute 85–90% of all cases of breast cancer *(JAMA 1999;281:2091–9)*.

In addition, a recent retrospective cohort study showed that women who use combination HRT have a greater breast cancer risk than those taking oestrogen alone *(JAMA 2000;283:485–91)*.

However, it is reassuring that five years after stopping HRT there is no longer an increased risk of breast cancer! There are further studies underway which will hopefully clarify the actual risk of breast cancer in women taking both opposed and unopposed oestrogens. The 'Million Women Study' was launched three years ago which aims to discover if HRT is linked to breast cancer. The Imperial Cancer Research Fund is funding the project which is involving 1 in 4 women aged between 50 and 64 years in the UK.

Does HRT offer protection against osteoporosis?
Numerous studies have shown that oestrogen reduces the risk of hip fracture by about 30% and of spine fracture by about 50%. The reduction in fracture risk by oestrogen exceeds that expected based on bone density alone. However, 10 years after HRT has been stopped, bone density and fracture risk are similar in women who have not taken HRT.

Do women taking HRT have a higher risk of deep vein thrombosis (DVT)?
The risk of DVT is very small in women taking HRT. Studies have shown that the absolute risk increases from 9 per 100,000 women in non-users to 30 per 100,000 in users.

Obstetrics & Gynaecology

Finally, the most commonly asked question by patients:

Does HRT cause women to put on weight?
Many women are worried about putting on weight when taking HRT. From many trials on HRT, however, it has been shown that all women put on weight after the menopause, but in general those taking HRT actually put on **less** weight than those in the placebo groups!

SUMMARY POINTS FOR HRT

- ❖ Association between HRT and CHD still controversial
- ❖ Risk of breast cancer in HRT users often over estimated
- ❖ Osteoporosis protection only when taking HRT
- ❖ Little evidence that HRT causes weight gain

CHAPTER 7: PAEDIATRICS

CHILDHOOD VACCINATIONS

Meningococcal C vaccination

The incidence of group C meningococcal infection has increased to account for approximately 40% of meningococcal disease. This rise is particularly prominent in teenagers, in whom mortality rates have been as high as 20%. It has been estimated that between July 1998 and June 1999 more than 1,500 cases of group-C disease occurred in the UK, leading to 150 deaths.

The new vaccine has an excellent safety profile in all ages and has been given to babies, young children, school-children and students. It has been estimated that since the launch of the vaccination just over a year ago, 500 cases of meningitis C and 50 deaths have been prevented. The Department of Health recently announced a 90% fall in the number of meningitis C cases in 15–17 year olds in the past six months compared with last year.

The Department of Health is currently investigating whether it is beneficial to give the vaccine to adults. A meningitis B vaccine is currently undergoing trials but is realistically several years away from a licence.

MMR vaccination

The uptake of the MMR vaccine in babies has reduced as a result of reports suggesting possible links with autism and inflammatory bowel disease. In some areas, the vaccination rates are now even below those needed to ensure herd immunity. There is concern that the incidence of measles and mumps is increasing as a result of this reduced uptake of the vaccination. As many as 1 in 4 four-year-olds in Surrey are currently unprotected.

Dr Andrew Wakefield has been at the forefront of suggesting the link between the MMR vaccine and long-term health problems, especially inflammatory bowel disease and autism. Media interest has also focussed on the use of single antigen vaccines as opposed to recommending the combined vaccine. There is real concern about having the vaccines separately, since children would then be left unnecessarily at risk from these potentially serious diseases. The problems with the studies were that they were all retrospective and so subject to recall bias by the parents and carers. The original studies also involved very small numbers of children.

Four independent bodies have reviewed the evidence: CSM, Joint Committee on Vaccination and Immunisation, MRC expert group and CSM Working Party on MMR Vaccine. They all agreed that the information does not support the suggested causal associations or give any cause for concern about the safety of the MMR vaccine. In addition, a very large Finnish study followed an impressive 1.8 million individuals for 14 years from the start of the MMR vaccination programme and it concluded that serious events are rare and are greatly outweighed by the risks of the disease. There were actually **no** cases of inflammatory bowel disease or autism detected in this study.

A recent study in London showed that although many mothers were influenced by the adverse media publicity, many mothers thought that the second dose of the MMR vaccine was unnecessary for their children. The majority of the 170 mothers said they valued their own GPs opinion the most when deciding whether to have their child vaccinated or not *(BGJP 2000;50:969–71)*. This is quite worrying as another study, which was based on 500 health care professionals, showed that almost half of GPs, health visitors and practice nurses felt very uneasy about giving the second dose of the MMR vaccine *(BMJ 2001;322:82–85)*. In addition, a third of the practice nurses thought that the link of the vaccine with Crohn's disease was either very likely or possible. This wide variation in knowledge regarding the vaccine may be influencing the advice that is given to parents.

 USEFUL WEBSITES

www.doh.gov.uk/mmrvac.htm – Department of Health site on MMR vaccination
www.immunisation.org.uk – NHS Health Promotion England immunisation website

---

SUMMARY POINTS ON MMR VACCINE

- ❖ Reduced uptake of vaccination
- ❖ MMR vaccine is very safe
- ❖ Wide variation in knowledge and attitudes amongst health care professionals
- ❖ Numerous incorrect media reports

Paediatrics

SUDDEN INFANT DEATH SYNDROME (SIDS)

The 'Back to Sleep' health education campaign has reduced the number of cot deaths in England and Wales from 1,000 to 400 a year.

Risk factors for SIDS include:
- Sleeping prone
- Male sex
- Parental smoking
- Previous SIDS in family
- Young maternal age
- Low socio-economic class
- High parity
- More occur in winter months

There are also some controversial risk factors. It was thought that mattress coverings containing fire retardant chemicals were associated with SIDS but these claims have been refuted. There is some evidence that breast feeding leads to a reduction in SIDS.

A recent three year study found that co-sleeping with an infant on a sofa is associated with a particularly high risk of SIDS. Bed sharing also increased the risk of SIDS if parents smoked, had recently drank alcohol, were excessively tired or had taken sedatives *(BMJ 1999;319:1457–62)*. Sharing a room with the parents was associated with a lower risk and it has even been recommended that parents should keep the child in their room for the first six months.

A recent study from Manchester showed a much higher presence of *Helicobacter pylori* in the tissue of SIDS babies compared with controls *(Arch Dis Child 2000;83:429–34)*. The sample size was very small and it may be an association rather than a direct cause of SIDS. However, it has been interpreted in the lay press that cot death could be passed to babies from parents and carers via their saliva from kissing their children!

 USEFUL WEBSITE

www.sids.org.uk/fsid – Sudden infant death syndrome website

CHAPTER 8: CANCER

THE NHS CANCER PLAN

The NHS Cancer Plan was introduced in September 2000. It is the first comprehensive national cancer programme and aims to improve the way in which cancer care is organised in the UK. It aims to:
* Save more lives
* Ensure cancer patients receive correct professional support and care
* Ensure patients receive the best available treatments
* Tackle the inequalities in cancer healthcare

The plan includes new targets for how quickly treatment should begin after patients see a consultant, and how soon treatment should begin after referral by a GP.

The Government believes that the targets can be met as it is proposing the creation of almost 1,000 new cancer consultant posts by 2006. The Government is also planning to increase investment in palliative care services and hospices by £50m; provide more treatment equipment and 250 new scanners.

Cancer specialists have already expressed doubts about whether the NHS would be able to achieve the targets that have been set *(BMJ 2000;321:850)*. They have welcomed the increased funding for cancer services but have said it is doubtful whether some of the targets could be met. For example, the target of a maximum two month wait from urgent GP referral to treatment for colorectal cancer may be unrealistic because presently the investigations necessary for a definite diagnosis can often take a month or more.

New targets to be introduced in stages
* Maximum 1/12 wait from urgent GP referral to treatment guaranteed for children's, testicular cancers and acute leukaemia by 2001
* Maximum 1/12 wait from diagnosis to treatment for breast cancer by 2001
* Maximum 1/12 wait from diagnosis to treatment for all cancers by 2005
* Maximum 2/12 wait from urgent GP referral to treatment for breast cancer by 2002

Cancer

- Maximum 2/12 wait from urgent GP referral to treatment for all cancers by 2005

How will the cancer plan affect GPs?

All primary care trusts will be expected to review their cancer screening coverage and improve the uptake, especially by ethnic minorities and deprived patient groups. A national system of cancer networks is being set up which aims to plan cancer services to meet individual needs and co-ordinate cancer plan initiatives at a local level. A lead clinician for cancer will be appointed for each primary care trust (PCT), this will be a GP who will have dedicated time to work for the cancer network and help to improve clinical standards. They will also help to improve communication across primary, secondary and tertiary services.

Cancer registers will also be established for each PCT and GPs will have to contribute to these. However, the GMC recently stated that consent from the patient is required before cancers can be registered which is likely to lead to chaos *(BMJ 2001;321:849)*. The UK Association of cancer registers have found that the most reliable and consistent data on cancers are obtained at time of diagnosis from histopathology departments – making consent very difficult. Patients must be given clear details on how the information from their disease may be used and they must have access to that information in order to be assured of its validity.

What role should GPs play in cancer diagnosis and treatment?

General Practitioners are gradually becoming more involved in managing patients with cancer. They are concerned with the comprehensive, co-ordinated and continuous care of individuals, families, and, increasingly, populations. General Practitioners have an important role in cancer management and the British Government's desire to improve cancer outcomes relies heavily on General Practitioners playing their part.

Diagnosing cancer in primary care is often difficult. Many cancers present with common symptoms such as persistent cough or non-specific abdominal pain yet few patients with such symptoms turn out to have cancer. Primary care clinicians need to be able to discriminate which patients within a relatively unselected population have a higher likelihood of malignant disease. The Government has produced guidelines regarding urgent referrals of patients with suspected malignancies and most hospital departments have created referral forms for GPs to complete as a consequence of these guidelines.

Cancer

What are the problems with the GP referral guidelines?
They have recently been criticised as they are based on poor-quality evidence; the evidence used was from patients seen in secondary and tertiary care and then applied to primary care. Many of the guidelines are quite general and it may be that the system becomes overloaded very quickly which would then be detrimental to cancer patients. For example, referral guidelines for upper gastrointestinal cancers have been introduced recently which state that 'all patients over the age of 55 years with symptoms which could be due to upper GI cancer must be seen within two weeks' – this surely will overwhelm already very stretched clinics!

How do GPs contribute to cancer screening?
General Practitioners occupy a critical position in ensuring the effectiveness of national cancer screening programmes as well as providing effective and cost-effective advice on specific primary prevention strategies. In the UK's breast and cervical cancer screening programmes primary health care team members have both developed and been delegated important roles in providing information and advice to women at all stages of the screening process *(BMJ 2000;320:1090–1)*.

Patients often do not understand the rationale for screening or the inevitability of some false positive and false negative results. General Practitioners thus have an important and expanding role in ensuring that their patients truly understand these issues and the need for continuing vigilance about new symptoms.

What are Wilson's criteria for screening?
These are well established criteria which should ideally be met before implementing a screening programme. They are important to know and can be applied to other screening programmes as well as to different types of cancer. There are, however, very few conditions for which all the criteria can be met.

They state that:
- The condition should be common and important
- There must be a latent period or early symptomatic stage during which effective treatment is possible
- There must be acceptable and available treatment for the disease
- The untreated natural history of the disease must be known
- The screening tests must be acceptable, cost-effective, safe and reliable

Cancer

- The screening test should be highly sensitive and specific
- The screening should be continuous (not just a 'one off' test).

What are the ethics of screening?
The four main principles of ethics should be applied here (they are very useful to know for the viva exam!): Beneficence (do good), Non-maleficence (do no harm), Autonomy and Justice.

- **Beneficence**
The benefit of screening must outweigh any potential harm to an individual.

- **Non-maleficence**
There are both personal costs and costs to society to consider. Personal costs include problems with false positive results, which can lead to distress and possible unnecessary treatment. No test is 100% specific. False negatives also can occur, as no test is 100% sensitive, which can then lead to false reassurance by both patients and doctors. This may even dissuade patients from returning for future screening tests.

Misinterpretation of results can lead to a false sense of security, for example patients with normal cholesterol or normal blood pressure may continue to smoke. The effects of the screening test itself need to be considered, for example, radiation exposure with X-rays. There are also the costs to society, for example, the actual costs of equipment, facilities, treatment, and also the time taken off work for people to attend the screening test and the treatment.

Finally, there are psychological costs involved, it is known that patients who have been diagnosed with a high blood pressure have higher rates of depression and lower self-esteem, even if they are later told that their blood pressure is normal.

- **Autonomy**
Many people believe it is their right to know what is going on in their body whereas others have different health beliefs and cultures and object to being screened. This needs to be respected when considering individual autonomy.

- **Justice**
Implementing screening tests may mean that funds are diverted from

Cancer

other services, for example cancer treatments. The correct allocation of limited resources is very important, especially in the current climate.

 USEFUL WEBSITE

www.doh.gov.uk/cancer

SUMMARY POINTS FOR CANCER

- Over-ambitious targets in NHS Cancer Plan
- Lead clinician to be appointed for each PCT
- GPs have a crucial role in both cancer and cancer screening
- Wilson's criteria should be met for screening programmes
- Consider the ethics of screening

Cancer

PROSTATE CANCER

Prostate cancer is a very common disease – the incidence is rising as a result of earlier detection of the disease and an ageing population. It is the second commonest male cancer and over the last 20 years death rates from the disease have doubled. Approximately 60% of patients in the UK have metastases at the time of their diagnosis. Despite considerable advances in the ability to detect and treat prostate cancer, there have been no significant corresponding decreases in morbidity and mortality in the UK. Conversely, in the USA, where prostate cancer screening with PSA testing widely occurs, prostate cancer mortality has fallen by almost 3% per annum for the past three years.

Prostate cancer is increasingly detected at an earlier stage by serum measurement of prostate specific antigen (PSA), however it is still highly debatable as to whether screening for prostate cancer is worthwhile.

What are the benefits of measuring PSA levels in patients?
Prostate specific antigen is probably the best available blood test for detecting any cancer, it still has somewhat limited specificity. Its value has been improved by techniques such as monitoring change in concentration with time (velocity), assessing concentration in relation to prostate volume and to age, and, most recently, measuring the free to total prostate specific antigen ratio (the lower the ratio the greater the chance of prostate cancer being detected by biopsy).

What are the problems with measuring PSA levels in patients?
Controversy continues about the treatment of apparently localised prostate cancer *(BMJ 2000;320:69–70)*. However, radical treatment is generally not justified in patients with a PSA concentration over 20 µg/l, as the tumour will often extend beyond the prostatic capsule. The grade of tumour and the life expectancy of the patient also influence the final decision. Patients with well-differentiated tumours may do well without treatment, whereas those with poorly differentiated tumours usually do badly. Most men have moderately well differentiated tumours and are likely to benefit from radical treatment if they have a life expectancy of >10 years.

Certain events can result in a transient change in the serum PSA level. For example it can fall after a long period of recumbency and can increase with prostatic biopsy, transrectal ultrasound and vigorous prostatic massage. However, a digital rectal examination alone does not appear to have any significant effect on the serum PSA level.

What is the optimal treatment for prostate cancer?

This is an area of great debate as there is still no clear agreement as to the optimal treatment *(BMJ 1999;318:299–300)*. A Government-funded trial is commencing which will investigate the best treatment option for men who are diagnosed with prostate cancer – watchful waiting, radical surgery or radiotherapy.

Should prostate cancer be screened for?

Media publicity and a heightened public awareness of prostate cancer have increased the profile of PSA screening. The question of whether screening should be implemented is still extremely debatable. Firstly, only a minority of cancers spread beyond the gland to cause disease and shorten life expectancy. In addition, curative treatments have major side-effects (e.g. impotence and incontinence).

A large £13m screening trial is currently underway by researchers in Sheffield, Bristol and Newcastle, involving 230,000 men aged 50–69 years. They will be invited for PSA testing, along with counselling at their GP practice. Those with raised PSA will be offered digital rectal examination and prostate biopsy. Those with prostate cancer will be randomised to one of three treatment groups. This trial will 'help to establish whether to introduce a screening programme for prostate cancer'.

The National Screening Committee has advised against screening as:
- Many subclinical cases would be detected
- Excess anxiety would result
- In many cases there would be no change in the overall outcome or treatment
- The PSA level cannot predict whether the cancer is indolent or aggressive
- PSA has a poor specificity
- There is still a lack of consensus regarding treatment for early disease
- Physical harm of prostate biopsies
- Some cancers detected may never present clinically

There are also strong arguments towards introducing a screening programme including:
- Men's autonomy
- PSA is a cheap and readily available test
- Screening may possibly be beneficial (lack of evidence of

Cancer

effectiveness does not prove ineffectiveness)
- May lead to detection of early, potentially curable cancers

The proof of the ability of PSA testing to reduce the disease-specific mortality of prostate cancer will be provided by randomised controlled trials, which are currently underway in both USA and Europe. Unfortunately, it will be many years before these results are available and, in the interim, doctors must act on the information that is currently available in the best interests of their patients. Patients must be informed of the pros and cons of PSA testing and also the implications of a positive result before having a PSA test performed.

SUMMARY POINTS FOR PROSTATE CANCER

- ❖ Incidence of prostate cancer is rising
- ❖ Screening may occur in future
- ❖ Controversial treatment options exist

CHAPTER 9: ANTIBIOTICS

ANTIBIOTIC RESISTANCE

- House of Lords Select Committee Report (1998) highlighted the problem of increasing antibiotic resistance
- Most antibiotic use is in two areas, in humans in the community and in animals for growth promotion and prophylaxis
- Estimated that up to 75% of antibiotic use is of questionable value
- Increasing resistance problems are probably related to the use of broad spectrum agents, such as cephalosporins and crowding of susceptible people (nursing homes)
- Veterinary and agriculture practice will also have to change in the light of these findings

The Standing Medical Advisory Committee Report
- Antimicrobial use is an important driving factor in the emergence of resistance
- Use antimicrobial agents prudently and keep unnecessary or inappropriate prescribing to the minimum
- Primary care accounts for 80% of antimicrobial prescribing in the UK

Recommendations:
National campaign should be launched to increase public and health professionals' understanding of the problem. Use of prescription guidelines.

Four areas have been identified that could make a significant impact on the volume of antimicrobials prescribed:
1. No prescribing of antibiotics for simple coughs and colds
2. No prescribing of antibiotics for viral sore throats
3. Limit prescribing for uncomplicated cystitis to 3 days in fit young women
4. Limit prescribing of antibiotics over the telephone to exceptional cases

In September 1999, the Government launched a national public education campaign (they used a character called 'Andy Biotic') on antibiotic resistance. It aimed to support health professionals in their management of patients with acute URTI by reducing patients expectations for antibiotics from their GP, and promoted seeking advice from community pharmacists.

Antibiotics

ANTIBIOTICS AND ACUTE OTITIS MEDIA

Definition: Otitis media is inflammation in the middle ear.

Subcategories include acute otitis media, otitis media with effusion (also known as 'glue ear'), recurrent acute otitis media and chronic suppurative otitis media. Acute otitis media presents with systemic and local signs and has a rapid onset. The persistence of an effusion beyond three months without signs of infection defines otitis media with effusion, whereas chronic suppurative otitis media is characterised by continuing inflammation in the middle ear giving rise to otorrhoea and a perforated tympanic membrane.

- Acute otitis media is a common condition with a high morbidity and low mortality
- In the UK about 30% of children aged under 3 years visit their GP with acute otitis media each year
- 97% receive antimicrobial treatment
- 1:10 children will have an episode of acute otitis media by 3 months of age
- Most common bacterial causes for acute otitis media are *Streptococcus pneumoniae*, *Haemophilus influenzae* and *Moraxella catarrhalis*
- Risk factors for poor outcome are young age and attendance at day care centres such as nursery schools
- Others risks include white race, male sex and history of enlarged adenoids, tonsillitis and asthma
- Factors predisposing to poor outcome: multiple previous episodes, bottle feeding, history of ear infections in parents or siblings and use of a soother/pacifier
- Evidence for the effect of environmental tobacco smoke is controversial
- In 80% of children the condition resolves without antibiotic treatment in about three days
- Complications are rare but include hearing loss, mastoiditis, meningitis and recurrent attacks
- In the developed world, the majority of children with acute otitis media are treated with antibiotics
- In the Netherlands only a minority are, but the outcome seems no worse
- Antibiotics give limited benefits
- Most children can be treated without antibiotics

Antibiotics

- Pain lasts no more than 24 hours in 80% of children
- Benefits of withholding antibiotics include reduced cost, reduced side-effects and reduced antibiotic resistance

'Clinical Evidence' published by the BMJ Publishing Group included a review of the effects of treatment for otitis media and of the effects of preventive interventions. This particular section also appeared in the BMJ (25 September 1999).

KEY POINTS FOR ACUTE OTITIS MEDIA

- Limited evidence from one RCT that non-steroidal anti-inflammatory drugs are more effective than placebo in relieving pain in children with acute otitis media
- Effectiveness of antibiotics is conflicting
- The review found no clear evidence favouring a particular antibiotic for acute otitis media
- One systematic review of RCTs found greater immediate benefit but no difference in long-term outcome with short (≤5 days) rather than longer courses of antibiotics
- One systematic review of RCTs has found that long-term antibiotic prophylaxis has a modest effect in preventing recurrences of acute otitis media. However, which antibiotic to use, for how long and how many episodes of acute otitis media justify treatment have not been adequately evaluated.

PAPERS:

 Del Mar
(BMJ 1997;314:1526–29)
Meta-analysis of controlled trials (antibiotics vs placebo):
- Early use of antibiotics conferred marginal benefit with 17 requiring immediate treatment to prevent one getting pain at 2–7 days
- Antibiotics benefit only those 14% still in pain 24 hours after presentation
- Antibiotics double the risk of vomiting, diarrhoea and rashes

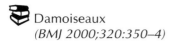 Damoiseaux
(BMJ 2000;320:350–4)

RCT of Amoxycillin vs placebo in under two-year-olds:
- Amoxycillin reduced duration of pain and fever by about one day
- No difference in outcome at 11 days
- Seven to eight need to be treated with antibiotic for one to benefit
- Very modest benefit does not justify treating every child with antibiotic
- Watchful waiting is justified

Suggested evidence-based management
Explain that:
- Most cases get better within 24 hours without antibiotics
- Most cases are due to viruses which are not killed by antibiotics
- Withhold antibiotics in mild cases
- Advise four hourly paracetamol in correct doses
- Offer to review child in 24–72 hours if parental/doctor concern
- Consider information leaflets
- Consider deferred prescription of antibiotic, only to be used if child is no better after 24–48 hours
- Consider antibiotic at outset if child is unduly ill, toxic or has a high fever

SORE THROAT

When should we use antibiotics?
Antibiotics have been used in the past in order to:
- Reduce severity or shorten duration of symptoms
- Reduce risk of complications, suppurative (quinsy, otitis media, sinusitis) and non-suppurative (rheumatic fever, nephritis)
- Satisfy non-clinical purposes such as perceived patient demand and terminating the consultation

But
- At least 70% of sore throats are caused by viruses
- We now have evidence to help us select those patients who probably have a bacterial infection and may benefit from penicillin

PAPERS:

 Penicillin for acute sore throat: randomised double-blind trial of 7 days vs 3 days treatment or placebo in adults.
(Zwart, BMJ 2000;320:150–4)
- GP based study from the Netherlands
- Randomised to penicillin V for 7 days, penicillin V for 3 days followed by placebo for 4 days or placebo for 7 days
- Sore throats for less than 7 days and with three of the four 'Centor' criteria:
  - Fever
  - No cough
  - Tonsillar exudate
  - Swollen, tender, anterior cervical nodes

Showed that penicillin V for seven days resulted in
- Two days shorter duration of symptoms
- Reduced incidence of complications (quinsy)
- Supports use of penicillin V in patient with three of the four 'Centor' criteria

Arguments against using an antibiotic
- Benefit shown is so modest that one can dispute its clinical importance
- Actual benefit is marginal/modest at best
- Harms may outweigh benefits. Bacterial resistance, allergic reactions (rashes/anaphylaxis 2-4:10,000 and death 2:100,000)
- Diarrhoea, candidiasis, unplanned pregnancy if on COCP

Antibiotics

- Costs to NHS
- Increased patient dependence, expectation and future demands

 Randomised trial of prescribing strategies in managing a sore throat.
(Little, BMJ 1997;314:722)

- Designed to test three different prescribing strategies in terms of duration of symptoms, satisfaction and compliance with treatment and time off school and work
- They were:
  1. 10 days prescription for antibiotics
  2. No prescription
  3. Prescription if symptoms did not settle in 3 days
- No significant difference in the proportion of patients better in 3 days, duration of illness, time to return to work or satisfaction
- More people in the first group thought antibiotics were effective and intended coming to the doctor in future attacks
- 69% of patients in the delayed prescription group did not use their prescriptions
- Concluded that antibiotics had a marginal clinical effect
- Prescription resulted in enhanced belief and intention to re-consult when compared to other groups

 Reattendence and complications in randomised trial of prescribing strategies for sore throat: the medicalising effects of antibiotics.
(Little, BMJ 1997;315:350–2)

- Aim to assess the medicalising effect of prescribing antibiotics
- Randomisation as above
- Outcome measures were number and rate of patients making a first return with sore throat, early return (within two weeks) and complications
- Followed up for 1 year, those initially prescribed antibiotics presented in a higher proportion within the year with sore throats
- Longer duration of illness also increased chance of return
- No difference between the various groups in terms of early return or complications
- Previous and current prescribing increases re-attendance

 Antibiotics for symptoms and complications of sore throat.
(Del Mar, The Cochrane Library, issue 2, 2001. Oxford: Update software)

Antibiotics

- Found that prescribing antibiotics reduced the symptoms of sore throat; fever and headache by 50% in the short-term, but 90% of all patients were symptom free by 1 week
- Due to pooling of data (large number of patients) rarer complication rates could be elicited
- Risk of rheumatic fever reduced by 30%, but unable to assess whether treatment offered protection against glomerulonephritis as numbers were still too small
- Effect of antibiotics on suppurative complications, acute otitis media reduced by 25%, acute sinusitis by 30% and quinsy by 20%
- Concluded that antibiotics offer a modest clinical benefit
- In the western world the small reduction in rheumatic fever and glomerulonephritis was not thought to be worth recommending the routine use of antibiotics in sore throats

Clinical and psychosocial predictors of illness duration from randomised controlled trial of prescribing strategies for sore throat. (Little, BMJ 1999;319:736)

- Providing patients with information about duration of illness can reduce expectation and reattendance
- Studied factors that affect duration of sore throat and assessed whether satisfaction with the consultation independently predicts duration of illness
- Patients recorded satisfaction with the consultation and how well their concerns had been dealt with after the consultation and kept a diary of symptoms until better
- Older patients (over 12 years), those with longer duration of illness before consultation, those with cough and those who were less satisfied were more likely to have prolonged course
- Most people (69%) had their concerns very well dealt with; this was a better predictor of whether patients were very satisfied than whether an antibiotic was prescribed
- Satisfaction was not predicted by any other variable
- This trial excluded very ill patients, so may have exaggerated findings
- Satisfaction with the consultation predicted duration of illness independently of potential confounding variables and was more closely related to effective doctor-patient communication than to prescription of antibiotics
- Doctors should elicit patients' concerns and consider counselling patients, particularly those at risk of prolonged illness

128

CHAPTER 10: CLINICAL GOVERNANCE

"Clinical governance is a system through which NHS organisations are accountable for continuously improving the quality of their services and safeguarding high standards of care and creating an environment in which excellence in clinical care will flourish."

All health organisations will have a statutory duty to seek quality improvement through clinical governance. Financial control, service performance and clinical quality should be fully integrated at every level. Clinical governance is the Government's concept of the boards of Trusts and PCGs being as responsible for clinical performance as they are for financial and legal performance.

Guidelines for standards expected from GPs will come from national bodies (NICE). At a local level, a senior GP member of the PCG board is responsible for clinical governance within that PCG. Each practice has a partner who is responsible for developing clinical governance within that practice.

What are the components of clinical quality?
- Professional performance (technical quality)
- Resource use (efficiency)
- Risk management (risk of injury or illness associated with the service)
- Patient satisfaction

Why is it needed?
- GP quality is too variable
- Patients have a right to expect greater consistency in access to and quality of, primary care services
- Patients need to be assured that their treatment is up to date, effective and is provided by GPs who keep apace of modern developments

In reality
- Doctors must take part in audit
- Leadership skills must be developed within clinical teams
- Evidence-based medicine must be practised
- Good practice must be disseminated
- Risk management procedures must be in place
- Adverse events must be detected and investigated
- Lessons learnt must be applied to clinical practice
- Poor performance must be recognised early and tackled promptly

Clinical Governance

How will it translate in PCGs?
- Each PCG has to nominate a senior professional to lead on clinical standards and professional development
- Each practice must have a named clinical governance lead responsible for liasing with the rest of the PHCT and with the PCG
- PCGs will expect peer pressure and support to improve the quality of care within the group, by ironing out unacceptable variations
- Health Authorities will expect PCGs and individual practices to implement the clinical governance agenda, but they seem to have no sanctions they can apply to recalcitrant GPs
- Within PCGs, joint clinical responsibility is now added to individual clinical responsibility
- By 2002, PCGs should be delivering measurable improvements against locally agreed milestones and targets
- Information on quality (audits) may become public and identifiable as lay members of PCG may demand it and other doctors may want it

Which external bodies have been established to assist local quality improvements?

National Institute for Clinical Excellence (NICE) gives guidance by:
- Appraisal of evidence
- Development and dissemination of audit methods
- Development and dissemination of guidelines
- Effectiveness bulletins

Commission for Health Improvement (CHI)
- Government quality watchdog
- Consists of GPs, community nurses and lay people
- Plan is that they will visit each PCG every 4 years
- Looks at clinical governance at PCG level
- Visits a random selection of practices
- A collaborative approach with groups not up to scratch
- Has the ability to report under performing health bodies to the Health secretary
- Tells us whether we are following guidance by:
  - Provider and service reviews
  - Performance indicators
  - Troubleshooting problem areas

Beacon practices
Practices that can demonstrate high quality practice in areas such as health improvement, fair access, effective delivery and improved patient care or experience.
- Receive £4000 per year
- Apparently open for 12 days a year to share and disseminate their good practice
- Risk of elitism

Conclusions
- The advent of clinical governance is a watershed in the history of General Practice
- Each GP is responsible for providing high quality care, auditing care, auditing standards of themselves and their colleagues in the PCG
- Clinical governance is a powerful tool for improving quality of care in General Practice
- Clinical governance is a means of maintaining quality assurance and accountability to the public
- May be our last chance for self-regulation

PAPERS:

The following papers although not essential to the exam would provide you with a more in-depth understanding of the practical problems facing General Practice in the current political climate. Often editorials such as those which appear in the BMJ can make interesting reading when considering particular topics, often thought provoking and written by peers they can provide an alternative view that reading studies in isolation may not. They are often also easier to read and well referenced – they can be a good place to start for some topics. The first three papers were part of a series of five, written to encompass clinical governance in practice.

 Clinical governance in primary care – Knowledge and information for clinical governance
(BMJ 2000;321:571–74)
This paper discussed the additional knowledge that will be required by all staff working in primary care and the challenges faced by leaders of primary care groups and trusts. They suggested where relevant information could be found. Everyone in primary care needs to be familiar with these sources if clinical governance is to succeed as a way to improve the quality of health care.

Clinical Governance

Summary points
- Everyone in primary care needs to be familiar with the requirements of clinical governance if it is to succeed as a way to improve the quality of care
- Producing, collecting and analysing primary care information is difficult, but some practices have already overcome these barriers
- Individuals and primary care group and trust leaders can do much to promote clinical governance, but problems remain

The version of this paper on the BMJ's website includes numerous URLs to show what information is available.

📖 Clinical governance in primary care: participating in clinical governance
(M Pringle, BMJ 2000;321:737–40)
Emphasised the need for clinicians to find information, which will improve their own practice and aid learning in the primary care team as a whole. Such work is likely to go a long way towards fulfilling the GMC's requirements for revalidation.

- NeLH (The National Electronic Library for Health) will eventually help to improve access to information in the practice. In one English region only 20% of GPs had access to bibliographic databases in their surgeries and 17% had access to the Internet
- Primary care groups and trusts will need to invest in adequate information technology hardware, software and training
- Avoid duplication of effort, relevant information should be co-ordinated at a national level and facilitated locally through postgraduate libraries
- Computerised clinical decision support systems used during consultations can help to improve performance and patient outcomes
- In England and Wales, Prodigy software is available free of charge on 85% of computer systems; it can offer advice during consultations on what to do in over 150 conditions commonly seen in primary care
- The MIQUEST project is one of the national facilitating projects within the NHS information management and technology strategy. It aims to help practices standardise their data entry and provides software to help with data extraction, including data required for national performance indicators.

Clinical Governance

 Accountability for clinical governance: developing collective responsibility for quality in primary care
(BMJ 2000;321:608–11)

This paper discussed how the notion of accountability in clinical governance could be understood and used within primary care.

- It will use the clinical governance work of a London PCG as a case study to illustrate mechanisms and different forms of accountability between health professionals
- Clinical governance will extend primary health care professionals' accountability beyond current forms of legal and professional accountability
- Clinical governance in primary care is aimed at enhancing the collective responsibility and accountability of professionals in primary care groups or trusts
- It is mainly concerned with increasing the accountability of primary health professionals to local communities (downwards accountability), the NHS hierarchy (upwards accountability) and their peers (horizontal accountability)
- Primary care groups and trusts may find that, in addition to encouraging a culture of accountability, financial incentives are useful to achieve greater accountability

 Using clinical evidence Barton, Editor for Clinical Evidence.
(BMJ 2001;322:503–4)

Points raised

- Most health carers want to base their practice on evidence and feel that this will improve patient care
- The original idea that each health professional should formulate questions themselves; search, appraise and summarise the literature and apply the evidence to patients has proved too difficult alongside the competing demands of clinical practice
- Over 90% of British GPs believe that learning evidence handling skills is not a priority and even when resources are available, doctors rarely search for evidence
- However, 72% often use evidence-based summaries generated by others, which can be accessed by busy clinicians in seconds
- The NHS will now be providing many of its clinicians with one of those sources of Clinical Evidence
- Clinical Evidence is a compendium of summaries of the best available evidence about what works and what does not work in health care

Clinical Governance

- It is constructed by transparent methods and updated regularly (so earlier issues should be discarded)
- In addition, NHS professionals in England and Scotland can access Clinical Evidence through the National Electronic Library for Health (NeLH) or through one of the 14,000 paper copies that are being distributed to NHS institutions
- Will the distribution of Clinical Evidence improve patient care? Sadly, there are no large studies of the results of distributing similar printed materials
- One systematic review (nine studies) found that the passive distribution of printed educational materials compared with no distribution produced only small effects of uncertain clinical importance
- Printed materials may be necessary to transmit knowledge but they are probably insufficient to change practice
- No study explored why printed materials were ineffective

It is not surprising that passive distribution of printed materials does not automatically change behaviour:
- Information may have been difficult to access when it was needed
- May have been difficult to understand or be irrelevant
- May have lacked credibility without a method of checking that the information is rigorous and complete

Clinical evidence presents the evidence but does not tell doctors or patients what to do because evidence is only part of making a clinical decision. Clinical expertise to evaluate each patient's circumstances and personal preferences is also important. Even the best available evidence may need adapting for individual patients. Thus a valid, relevant and accessible source of detailed clinical evidence is a necessary but not sufficient precursor of innovation to achieve evidence-based health care. Additional professional, educational and operational support for clinical innovation will probably accelerate the use of clinical evidence. Clinical Evidence will provide access to evidence in the way that the BNF provides access to prescribing information and earn as welcome a place in the consulting room.

134

CHAPTER 11: REVALIDATION

The Government has become increasingly concerned about the profession's ability to hold on to self-regulation. Much of the criticism has been aimed at the GMC. The public has also, through the Bristol case, Shipman and others, lost its faith in the GMC. At the BMA conference (2000) doctors passed a no confidence motion in the GMC. The GMC is currently undergoing a period of reform to try to convince all three parties that it is fit to continue to regulate the profession. One of the most important areas that the GMC will be judged upon is the introduction of revalidation.

Self-regulation
- 'A privilege, not a right' whereby the profession determines its own training, qualifications and codes of ethics and behaviour
- Threatened by recent events causing:
    - Loss of confidence by public
    - Perception that profession closes ranks to protect own interests
- Demands for greater transparency and accountability
- Undermined by less deferential and better informed public

Arguments for self-regulation
- Doctors' performance can be judged adequately only by someone doing the same job
- Self-regulation engenders self respect and motivation to perform well
- Self-regulation helps maintain professionalism and gives doctors a direct interest in maintaining standards
- Without self-regulation, doctors would cease to be a profession

Organisation of self-regulation
- GMC currently consulting with the profession, the public and the Government
- GMC wants all doctors to demonstrate competence at regular intervals by means of 'revalidation'
- Specialists place on Specialist Register may be made dependent on revalidation
- GMC may create a 'Generalists Register' for GPs with inclusion dependent on revalidation
- Mechanism of revalidation to be supportive, not punitive and largely by peer review, not examination
- Poor performance must be recognised early and intervention must be sympathetic but decisive

Revalidation

- Support/retraining for under-performing doctors must be available
- Removal from Register to be used as last resort, only for those beyond help
- Overall, self-regulation must be robust and open to scrutiny, to avoid accusations of professional protectionism

Revalidation (reaccreditation)
- Inevitable if self-regulation is to survive
- Political pressure
- Managerial demands
- Patient expectations
- Professional acceptance

Risks
- Further controls lead to reduced morale
- Maintaining standards becomes following fashion
- Health Authority take over - run by managers and lay people, dominated by expectations of purchaser
- Possible inability to withstand legal challenge
- Possible deterioration into an empty chore diverting doctors' time and energy from care of patients

Preferred scenario
- Professionally controlled
- Education-led (not examination-driven)
- Performance-based (e.g. peer review, audit, self-appraisal, patient satisfaction surveys)
- Help for under-performers
- Protected time
- New money to finance scheme

GMC Statement 1998
- Doctors in all disciplines must be able to show on a regular basis and throughout their careers, that they are keeping up-to-date and remain fit to practice
- Revalidation Steering Group to be set up to propose appropriate mechanisms
- GMC accepts principle of revalidation and will consult with the profession, the public and the Government on the mechanism
- Examination is inappropriate - revalidation should reflect performance at work
- Adequate resources will be needed

Revalidation

- RCGP to advise GMC on criteria and standards for General Practice
- Revalidation will involve local delivery of a system based on national standards, with transparency for the public, employers and the profession

Revalidation for Clinical General Practice
The RCGP established a Revalidation Working Group who produced this document for discussion by the profession. Details of the process of revalidation are yet to be announced.

The working group identified the following criteria to assess a system of revalidation – it should:
- Be understood by the public and be credible
- Identify unacceptable performance
- Identify good performance
- Be supported by the profession and support the profession
- Be practical and feasible
- Not put any particular group of practitioners at an advantage or a disadvantage

GPC/RCGP revalidation criteria
GPs will have to show that they:
- Are keeping up-to-date
- Are competent
- Prescribe cost-effectively
- Possess appropriate diagnostic and treatment equipment
- Keep up-to-date, accurate and legible records
- Are able to work in teams
- Have a satisfactory complaints procedure
- Respond rapidly to emergencies
- Have opening times that meet the needs of patients
- Set aside time for receiving and returning calls
- Listen to patients and explain management
- Know their professional limits

Revalidation

GMC proposals for revalidation May 2000

They see the benefits of revalidation:

For Patients	For Doctors	For Employers
Protecting them from poorly performing doctors	Helping conscientious doctors to show that they are giving good medical care	Providing the assurance and protection that will flow from knowing that the doctors they employ are fit to practice
Promoting good medical practice	Enabling doctors to correct weaknesses in their practice	Providing additional mechanisms to identify poor performance
Making the register a valid indicator of current fitness to	Protecting doctors from unfounded criticisms of their	

GPs will have to compile a personal revalidation folder to include
- Personal information and CV and details of type of practice. Information about performance, this should be collected against each of the headings of Good Medical Practice. Details of any patient complaints and compliments, critical incidents and continuing professional development.
- A personal action plan of training and remedial action of problem areas, including the timescale for improvement
- This folder will probably be appraised on an annual basis with another medical practitioner who is professionally accountable to the GMC. A revalidation group will then perform an assessment of the folder every five years and recommend whether the doctor is revalidated or referred to the GMC.
- As part of clinical governance, doctors will need to have a personal development plan which will form the central component of revalidation

Revalidation

Current Situation

 Assuring the quality of medical practice, implementing 'Supporting doctors, protecting patients'
(January 2001. The latest report from the DoH regarding revalidation.)

Key recommendations
- A new National Clinical Assessment Authority to assess poorly performing doctors by practice visits
- Annual appraisals for all GPs to start from 2001 (delayed to 2003 at time of going to press)
- First decisions on GP revalidation in 2003
- A revised national disciplinary procedure for GPs
- Pre-employment checks to be introduced in 2001
- Guidance for a new occupational health service in 2001
- A new independent patient advocacy service to help patients with complaints against doctors

Patient power
- New national network of patient forums to monitor health organisations, supported by a Patient Advocacy and Liaison Service (PALS)
- Separate independent patient advocacy service to help with complaints
- NHS organisations to produce patient prospectuses to report action on patients' comments
- A local authority scrutiny committees to monitor HAs
- A more patient-friendly complaint system expected after DoH review

Discipline and GMC
- Revised disciplinary action
- Revised suspension action
- Alert letters to warn about bad doctors
- GMC future rests with Government
- GMC civil burden of proof to make it easier to strike off doctors
- Council to become part of UK Council of Health Regulators

Revalidation

Performance
- Annual appraisal for all doctors including locums to begin this year
- All doctors to carry out medical audits
- New systems to report adverse incidents, feeding into a national register
- National Clinical Assessment Authority to deal with poor and under-performing doctors

Other key points
- National Clinical Governance Support Team set up in 1999 to become part of the Modernisation Agency
- Information technology implications of NHS plan due 2001
- New pre-employment checks for primary care to be introduced 2001
- New guidance on occupational health service due 2001

Statutory changes
- GPs to declare criminal convictions
- Mandatory exclusion from HA lists for murder. Other convictions at HA discretion.
- HAs to keep list of locums, deputies and assistants
- Immediate suspension from HA list if there are patient safety fears
- Only GPs on HA list can practise
- Deaths in surgery to be reported
- GPs to declare all gifts

National Clinical Assessment Authority
- From April 2001 will offer a rapid performance, assessment and support service for doctors
- To recommend monitoring, education, retraining, medical treatment or referral to the GMC
- Special HA status
- HA can refer doctors for advice and assessment
- Assessment carried out via practice visits
- HA will still be able to refer to GMC or deal with doctor directly
- Assessors will be lay and medical
- GPs will be able to self refer
- NHS pays for assessment
- GPs will have input
- Links with postgraduate deans and tutors
- Disciplinary action if GPs refuse to co-operate

Revalidation

PRACTICE AND PERSONAL DEVELOPMENT PLANS

Response to criticism that PGEA (Postgraduate Education Allowance) is based on didactic, top-down, unprofessional model of CME. Criticisms of CME:

- GPs have gone on courses not related to the skills or knowledge that would benefit the practice population
- Rarely involves whole practice team
- Shows little evidence of producing changes in behaviour, organisational improvements, or benefits to patient care
- Provides convenient marketing opportunities to pharmaceutical industry

Thus, greater co-ordination between educational needs and service delivery is needed. The Government paper *'A first class service'*, supports the identification of professional and service needs in personal and practice development plans. The PDP will also be the basis on which revalidation and annual appraisal is based, so avoid them at your peril!

Aims

- Combine personal self-directed learning with organisational development framework
- To predispose to, enable and reinforce change, i.e. deliver information, rehearse behaviours, provide reminders and feedback
- Require learning portfolios for all members of practice team (doctors, nurses, managers), taking into account development needs of both individuals and the working unit
- Involve shift away from individual performance to organisational performance as measure of quality
- Patient involvement should ensure local responsiveness and prevent loss of personal care

Benefits include

- Teamwork to set and deliver priorities
- Systems to measure achievement of priorities
- Lever for change in primary care
- Greater personal and professional satisfaction
- More relevant to personal needs
- More flexible
- Aids reflection
- Recognises all the learning undertaken
- Freedom from the PGEA points scramble

Revalidation

- Fulfils Government and professional requirements
- Improves patient care
- Makes us more cost effective

Unresolved problems include
- Funding for plans involving several disciplines
- Accreditation for plans involving several disciplines
- Structure to facilitate, maintain and appraise

Revalidation

PRACTICE PROFESSIONAL DEVELOPMENT PLANS (PPDPs)

Ask yourself
- What do we need to do to improve our own practice?
- How have we identified what we need to do?
  - Discussions
  - Surveys
  - Audits
  - Significant event analysis
- Are these needs specific to our own practice, or do they reflect priorities in our PCG, Health Authority or the wider NHS?
- How are we going to address these needs?
- How will we judge our success?

Personal Development Plans (PDPs)

Ask yourself
- What do I need to do to improve the quality of care I provide? ('Reflection')
- How can I achieve these aims? ('Education')
- You choose your education on the basis of what you need to learn. (Continuous professional development (CPD))
- The **Johari Window** can provide a helpful model that can be used to remember the different techniques and people who can help.

  1. Keep a problem list for one month of subjects or issues you have found difficult
  2. Review your referral letters for one month
  3. Look at audits performed over the last year
  4. Reflect on the past month
  5. Use your clinical governance report as a source of learning needs!
  6. Try to identify the hidden needs by asking partners, staff, patients, nurses, family and friends. Also use of video work on improving technique.
  7. Critical incidence reporting

A PDP is part of the PPDP, as the team (practice) may require an individual to learn new skills in order to develop services.

143

Thus:
There is a lot in common between Clinical Governance (CG) and PPDPs/PDPs. Education should help you maintain and improve the quality of your care.

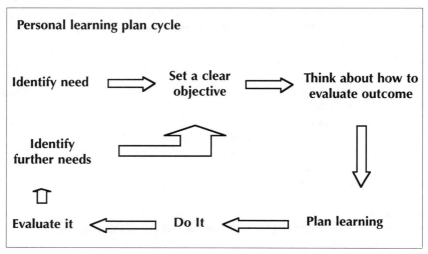

Risks of self-directed learning
- Self-directed learning can lead to isolation
- Lack of objectivity may lead to standards slipping
- May become overwhelmed and lose heart
- To help keep motivated, many self-directed learners use support networks including mentors
- A mentor is someone who can help you to learn more effectively, with whom you can share experiences and who will help you reflect on them and plan your next steps

The Learning Portfolio

Contains
- All past significant sources and experiences of learning
- May include a description of your work and practice
- A summary of all your learning experiences
- A description of how you would like to develop professionally in the future
- Personal development plan would be at the heart of the learning portfolio

Revalidation

- Portfolio would act as a more long-term record of past experience and future aspirations

Could include
- Workload logs
- Case descriptions
- Videos
- Audits
- Patient surveys
- Research projects
- Accounts of change or innovations
- Reflective diaries on study and ongoing education

CHAPTER 12: THE FUTURE OF GENERAL PRACTICE

Current problems
- Job satisfaction
- Morale
- Autonomy
- Workload
- Bureaucracy
- Recruitment
- Retention

GP numbers threatened by
- More early retirement
- More part-time principals/women principals (career breaks)
- More doctors needed in secondary care
- Reduced immigration from outside EU

Possible solutions
- Increased medical school intake
- Increased resources for staff premises and technology
- Increased delegation to Practice Nurses (Nurse Practitioners)
- Limiting expansion of GP workload, especially from secondary to primary care
- Core contract changed to ensure GPs retain control of workload (variable, flexible, minimal, practice based rather than individual)
- Appropriate funding for care transferred from secondary to primary care
- Easier re-entry arrangements after a career break
- Flexible working arrangements
- Increased linking of practices through PCGs, PCTs and Co-operatives
- Other health care professionals working in surgeries, e.g. pharmacists, physiotherapists, chiropractors, osteopaths, social workers, optometrists
- GPs employed by Community Trusts
- Initial triage by Nurse Practitioners - GP becomes specialist in family medicine (i.e. team leader) to be called only when needed
- Split contract - day and night elements

The Future of General Practice

THE NHS PLAN

The National Plan for the NHS, published in 2000, is the Government's vision for the NHS. This is a plan for investment in the NHS with sustained increases in funding. The purpose and vision of this NHS Plan is to give the people of Britain a health service fit for the 21st century: a health service designed around the patient. Public consultation for the Plan showed that the public wanted to see:
- More and better paid staff using new ways of working
- Reduced waiting times and high quality care centred on patients
- Improvements in local hospitals and surgeries

In summary, the aims:

Patients	Delivering fast and convenient care. Listening to their needs and letting them know their rights.
Professions	The entire NHS work force must work together to deliver services for patients. More co-operation between health care professionals.
Performance	Set and deliver high standards in the NHS.
Prevention	Promote healthy living across all sections of society. Deal with regional variations in care.
Partnership	Working together across the NHS to ensure the best possible care.

General Practice
More expansion to Personal Medical Services (PMS) is planned. New contractual quality standards for single-handed practices through a re-negotiated red book or a national PMS contract.

- Annual appraisals and audits will be mandatory
- Extension of nursing and other roles - by 2004 more than half of nurses will be able to prescribe medicines
- Practice referrals will be monitored
- Prescribing incentives will be offered by April 2001

Investment
- 7,000 extra beds in hospitals and intermediate care
- Over 100 new hospitals by 2010 and 500 new one-stop primary care centres

147

The Future of General Practice

- Over 3,000 GP premises modernised and 250 new scanners
- Clean wards – overseen by 'modern matrons' – and better hospital food
- Modern IT systems in every hospital and GP surgery
- 7,500 more consultants and 2,000 more GPs
- 20,000 extra nurses and 6,500 extra therapists
- 1,000 more medical school places
- Childcare support for NHS staff with 100 on-site nurseries

Reform
- New relationship between the DoH and the NHS to enshrine the trust that patients have in front-line staff
- A new system of earned autonomy will devolve power from the Government to the local health service as modernisation takes hold
- DoH will set national standards, matched by regular inspection of all local health bodies by an independent inspectorate, **CHI**
- **NICE** will ensure that cost-effective drugs like those for cancer are not dependent on where you live
- **The Modernisation Agency** will be set up to spread best practice
- Local NHS organisations that perform well for patients will get more freedom to run their own affairs
- There will also be a £500m performance fund
- But the Government will intervene more rapidly in those parts of the NHS that fail their patients

Integration
- Social services and the NHS will come together with new agreements to pool resources
- New Care Trusts to commission health and social care in a single organisation
- Modern contracts for both GPs and hospital doctors
- Extension of quality-based contracts for GPs in general and for single-handed practices in particular
- Consultants entitled to additional discretionary payments will rise from half to two-thirds but in return they will be expected to increase their productivity while working for the NHS
- Newly qualified consultants will not be able to do private work for perhaps seven years?

The Future of General Practice

Extended roles
- By 2004 over half of nurses will be able to supply medicines. £280m is being set aside over the next three years to develop the skills of staff.
- All support staff will have an Individual Learning Account worth £150 per year
- Number of nurse consultants will increase to 1,000 and a new role of consultant therapist will be introduced
- Leadership Centre will be set up to develop a new generation of managerial and clinical leaders, including modern matrons with authority to get the basics right on the ward

Patient power
- Letters about an individual patient's care will be copied to the patient
- Patients' views on local health services will help decide how much cash they get
- Patient advocates will be set up in every hospital
- If operations are cancelled on the day they are due to take place the patient will be able to choose another date within 28 days or the hospital will pay for it to be carried out at another hospital of the patient's choosing
- Patients surveys and forums to help services become more patient-centred

Recruitment
- By 2004 patients will be able to have a GP appointment within 48 hours
- Up to 1,000 specialist GPs taking referrals from fellow GPs
- Long waits in Accident and Emergency Departments will be ended
- By end of 2005 the maximum waiting time for an outpatient appointment will be three months and for inpatients, six months

Chronic diseases
- A big expansion in cancer screening programmes
- End to the postcode lottery in the prescribing of cancer drugs
- Rapid access chest pain clinics across the country by 2003
- Shorter waits for heart operations
- Hundreds of mental health teams to provide an immediate response to crises

Elderly
- Nursing care in nursing homes will be free
- By 2004 a £900m package of new intermediate care services to allow older people to live more independent lives
- National standards for caring for older people to ensure that ageism is not tolerated
- Breast screening to cover all women aged 65 to 70 years
- Personal care plans for elderly people and their carers

National inequalities target
- Increase and improve primary care in deprived areas
- Introduce screening programmes for women and children
- Step up smoking cessation services
- Improve the diet of young children by making fruit widely available in schools for 4–6 year olds

The summary and full document can be found on the internet:

 www.nhs.uk/nhsplan

 Shaping tomorrow: issues facing General Practice in the new Millennium GPC 2000

This was a discussion document issued by the General Practitioners Committee (GPC) of the BMA; it gathered views from the profession, politicians and patients. Each sub-heading below is an area discussed by the three parties. The salient points have been summarised. (This was a 80 page document – you're welcome to read all of it!).

My doctor or any doctor quickly
- Two apparent patient groups exist. The first group are essentially well and value easy access to health care with staff able to deal with their problem. The other are the chronically ill (elderly, poor) who place high value on seeing their doctor.

Divisions exist between GPs
- Some feel GPs over-invest in the notion of personal doctoring, like some psychological comfort blanket
- The personal relationship is something that many patients rate very highly
- Many GPs see the personal relationship as central to what they do

The Future of General Practice

- Others see it as a fading asset in a world of portfolio careers and part-time working
- A small minority, think the concept is dead and the profession should be honest that the future is increasingly likely to be about 'one hit' consultations
- Advocates of personal lists point out that knowledge of the patient reduces expenditure (fewer investigations etc.)

The RCGP Chairman Mike Pringle admits that in reality doctors are not able to provide continuity of care in their practice. GPs are increasingly being asked to do things that the Government (and some doctors) think is valuable, such as sit on PCG boards, organise education, do research, all of which means that they are not seeing patients. Other doctors (and the Government) feel that continuity of care is not as important an issue as the continuity of patient record. Some consensus exists that a core group of chronically ill patients benefit from having their own doctor and that this should always be a priority. The demands of the well population must not be allowed to overshadow the demands and needs of the chronically unwell.

The consultation is all? Or letting go to gain a richer day?
- Tensions exist between the call to reduce workload and to free up more time for longer consultations
- Some fear that giving up seeing some patients will reduce the quality of care, status or even pay
- Studies show that most patients are happy to see a nurse for triage/treatment of minor illness
- Opposing view is that there is no such thing as a minor illness or a trivial consultation. Each consultation is an opportunity for identifying the hidden agenda and that only someone sufficiently trained (GPs) will be able to uncover it.
- Evidence is scanty that an enormous increase in nurse care will reduce the utilisation of doctors (as in the US)
- Further research into the cost effectiveness of nurse practitioners is needed to see if indeed reduces the doctor's workload

Independent contractor status versus salaried service: phoney war or real debate?
The arguments for and against overlap, but essentially could be summed up as philosophical, clinical and financial – a heady enough mix to fuel any debate.

The Future of General Practice

Pros to IC status	Cons to IC status
• Allows GPs greater control of their jobs, (i.e. ways of working, hours, staff etc)	• Young doctors don't want to buy into partnerships
• Allows GPs to believe themselves to be other than 'mere employees of the state'	• Young Doctors want a more flexible way of working
• Allows GPs to be independent advocates on behalf of patients	• Perverse financial incentives, whereby a high list size and lack of investment in facilities and staff produces a better income than services provided by more conscientious GPs
• Allows innovation, promotes entrepreneurial spirit, encourages change and efficiency	• Researchers and academics complain of a data black hole in General Practice
• Leads to the development of vocational training, primary care teams, out-of-hours care and models of commissioning	• Much of the independence is illusory and will become more so in the future in a world of clinical governance, CHI, NSF, PCTs
• It is a cheap service	• A salaried system might stop
GPs	
• If all GPs were salaried and employed and therefore clocked on at 9 and off 36 hours later we would need far more GPs	worrying about money and allow them to get on with doctoring
	• Independent contractor status has at its heart a lack of

A job for life or portfolio careers

It isn't just changing patient expectations that will affect the shape of tomorrow's primary care – it is changing expectations among tomorrow's GPs. If young doctors want part-time working, flexible careers, the chance to move practices every few years and the opportunity to mix General Practice with other kinds of employment, then ultimately these desires need to be accommodated. It is undoubtedly tempting for an older generation of GPs to complain about 'Generation-X slackers'. There is a growing feminisation of the workforce, which raises issues about career breaks for motherhood and part-time working and perhaps leads to wider questions about public and political perceptions of General Practice in the future.

Failure to recognise and to respond to these risks is under-using a considerable resource; female doctors, ethnic minority doctors and non-principals in particular. This way of working will be better accommodated under a salaried, rather than premises-owning independent contractor partnerships. PMS pilots explore different ways of providing primary care – and are heavily supported in the NHS plan/Government.

NHS Direct and walk-ins: will they change the game?
More access points now exist – NHS direct, walk-in centres. Direct access to specialist care is expensive (but specialist GPs may be cheaper?). Those supporting NHS Direct and walk-ins believe they will work to reduce trivial demands on the time of GPs. Replacing phone calls to a surgery with a more systematic service, with quality assurance protocols, doesn't seem to pose a threat to General Practice. It seems to be potentially of considerable benefit. This Government is encouraging self-care and this has the capacity to benefit GPs. However, there is an unreasonable fear and paranoia about walk-in centres. There are something like 38 being established at present. Even if there were 60 or 70 or 400, you have to think of the numbers. If 100 centres treated 100,000 people a year that would be 10 million consultations. But there are 300 million patient contacts a year in General Practice. Nurses are also convinced that the service can help reduce unnecessary work for GPs, without undermining their position in primary care.

Clinical autonomy, does it have a place anymore?
In a world of NICE, NSF, guidelines and protocols, Prodigy, clinical governance and CHI does the concept of clinical autonomy have any real meaning anymore? Does this mean that GPs will lose the ability to mould care and treatment to individual patients? Many GPs take the view that guidelines and protocols are counsels of perfection, which are unobtainable under current resources, yet doctors (rather than politicians) will be held to account, when it is not possible to deliver services to such standards.

The Future of General Practice

Revalidation, poor performance, Bristol, are all saying to doctors 'you had better conform to the written standards otherwise you are out'. But if they do this it will produce huge cost pressures on the NHS. It is only because we use our generally excellent clinical judgement to flout almost every guideline going that this hasn't happened. Politicians are getting away with the rhetoric of perfection and doctors are being held to account for not delivering it.

Primary care groups: working together or professional straitjacket?

Will primary care groups, or trusts as they will eventually become, encourage GPs to work together in a more collective and co-operative way, or will they emerge as new bureaucracy imposing a deadening uniformity and extinguishing innovation and diversity? Alongside new structures there is a new public mood, which is demanding greater accountability from doctors and a more transparent understanding of how they arrive at the judgements they do and what yardsticks are used in these decisions. In a narrow sense it is not immediately clear to whom PCGs or PCTs will be accountable. The health authority? The NHS Executive? Ultimately to the Secretary of State, of course, but what will that mean for democracy on the ground?

In the wider sense of accountability, how will family doctors make it clear they want a genuine partnership with patients and are prepared to explain, and justify, what they do?

One of the hypotheses on which PCGs are based is that if you get doctors working in a more collaborative way you will then institute more peer comparison, peer review and ultimately more peer pressure to improve performance. On the other hand it is also a very clever political ploy to give clinicians an essentially inadequate unified budget and leave to them the impossible decisions regarding its distribution. GPs will need to decide how much they feel that they are acting in the patient's best interests by using their local and medical knowledge to distribute resources or whether they are compromising their role as the patient's advocate by becoming responsible for effectively rationing resources.

Accountability

Mike Pringle believes the profession is drinking in the last chance saloon when it comes to self-regulation and unless accountability is improved this will increasingly be imposed from outside by the Government.

If GPs don't do it themselves soon they are going to end up with a system

154

The Future of General Practice

of external regulation. A system of self-regulation needs to be put into place, which is there on the streets for everybody. Most doctors want to be good doctors and have a strong internal need to feel good about work *(hopefully)*. Nobody wants to do a bad job, although some people get themselves trapped. That professional drive needs to be valued.

Promoting Quality – what makes a good GP?

Is it possible that doctors, patients and politicians have different visions of what constitutes a quality service and, if so, how can these be reconciled? Among the mechanisms due to be launched to shore up quality, revalidation is the profession's own answer to charges that self-regulation is no longer up to the job of protecting the public. But will it work, or just be another burden GPs have to attend to every five years then forget about? If it is not to be too onerous and time-consuming, diverting resources from patient care, revalidation must judge with a fairly light hand, but will the public believe it has any validity?

Amongst many questions about how General Practice develops in the future is the issue of the generalist versus the sub-specialist. The generalist role is very dear to the heart of most GPs and is perhaps gaining increasing importance with the demise of the generalist hospital physician.

But many GPs also have special interests and would argue that such interests increase intellectual stimulation and allow GPs to better serve their patients. Should such interests and expertise be further formalised and made available not just within a practice but also between practices or even across a PCG?

What do patients want?

It is an old joke, but it still raises a smile at every medical retirement party. When asked what was the best part of the job, the GP always says 'the patients'. Asked next what was the worst thing about the job, the GP always replies 'the patients'. If the GP obtains intellectual stimulation from solving a medical jigsaw puzzle, or boosts his or her inner psyche by feeling they are contributing to a kinder world or making a difference, or even saving life, that's fine. But the patient just wants to get better. So what should the relationship of the future be between GPs and patients? Everyone talks of partnership and the end of benign paternalism, and patient autonomy and shared care, but it is not hard to feel sometimes that the profession looks over its shoulder and rather wishes that 'doctor knows best' was still a politically correct option.

If we are moving into a more honest and sharing relationship with patients, when doctors are advisers and guides and not gurus and wizards, there still seem few clear mechanisms to listen to what patients actually want, as opposed to doctors assuming they know what patients want. If patients become clients, or even customers, does that make doctors therapists and shopkeepers? And if it does, is that a bad thing?

What do patients want?
Claire Rayner, of the Patients' Association, firmly believes that the way forward is for the profession to see that patients are part of the health team and are as much involved with the provision, design, delivery and cost of health care as anyone else. She also recognises that because patients are recipients it does not alter the fact they have responsibilities to the service. But better ways of listening are needed. Patient liaison groups, citizen's juries and patient advisory panels seem to be the road we are going down. We do need much better mechanisms to get to hear the voice of the patient. GPs can't carry on being paternalistic. The days of a submissive, subdued, semiliterate, lumpen proletariat, people who were underfed, had rotten lives of quiet desperation, are over.

Funding and rationing – How is it all going to be paid for?
Most GPs would welcome a system that takes them out of the rationing front-line, be it a national rationing council, the Department of Health, or NICE. At the very least many would welcome a little more political honesty about the current situation. Proponents of the co-payment system argue that it would not only boost income for the health service, but also reduce workload. The counter-argument, of course, is that if people pay they become more demanding.

The Future of General Practice

'THE NEW NHS' (1997 Government white paper)

- 10 year programme of evolution rather than revolution
- Competitive internal markets to be replaced by co-operative integrated care (i.e. Partnership driven by performance)
- Purchaser-provider split for hospital care to continue
- Local doctors, nurses and health authorities to have new powers to commission services according to needs of patients
- NHS overhead costs to be cut, saving £1 billion in next five years
- Health Authorities to have greater supervisory role but will devolve responsibility for commissioning services to Primary Care Group
- NHS trusts to remain in present role as providers, but accountable to NHS regional offices, and required to publish costs of treatment to expose inefficiency
- Fundholding Scheme, which will be abolished from 1999 and replaced by Primary Care Groups
- Primary Care Groups, comprising all GPs and community nurses in an area, will commission health care for about 100,000 patients each
- Commission for Health Improvement will oversee quality of clinical services in NHS
- National Institute of Clinical Excellence will promote cost-effectiveness
- Telephone help line – NHS Direct – will advise patients on self-treatment 24 hours per day
- Local Health Improvement Programmes will monitor, plan and improve health care locally
- Advisory Committee on Resource Allocation will distribute NHS funds more fairly
- Annual survey of patients and users experience will compare performance
- Task force will involve NHS staff in planning the service

The Future of General Practice

RATIONING

Think of examples of scenarios where rationing may affect your practice, moral obligations, duty of care, post-code prescribing etc. For example Sildenafil (Viagra).

- Where in your practice do you prescribe to certain patients because of cost and not doubt over clinical efficacy?
- Rationing is regarded by many as the method by which the NHS might survive whilst delivering an apparently high standard of free quality care to the masses
- Can we continue to offer a gold standard free care as well as comprehensive care or are the two subject to financial forces?
- With rationing you could either deliver the 'best to most' or the 'average to all' what choice would you make?
- The general consensus is that the 'best to most' strategy is the best solution whilst maintaining a honesty and transparency to the public
- Politicians are unlikely to make this a public issue whilst trying to win elections, the stark reality that widespread rationing exists has rarely been admitted to and would ruffle many a feather

This problem has been actively explored in other countries. In 1993 'The Oregon Experiment' took place in the USA. Discussed in detail in an Education & Debate article in the BMJ *(1998;316:1965)*. A decade ago the state of Oregon attracted world-wide interest when it began an ambitious attempt to set priorities for health care on a systematic basis. Stimulated by the death of a 7-year-old boy who had been waiting for a bone marrow transplant operation, and led by John Kitzhaber, a doctor turned politician, Oregon passed legislation in 1989 designed to provide access to health insurance for all residents.

This was a huge market research exercise, which gathered opinions from a broad public base, treatments were explained and justified and a list was compiled according to priority. Compilation of the list included a weighting to clinical effectiveness, social values and emphasis on primary/preventative care. The difference was that the information gathered was used; a cut off line for conditions to be funded was decided according to available resources but remained dynamic with regular review.

In New Zealand, a Government appointed committee made a broad assessment of treatment priorities, as in the US, involving the public. It

158

The Future of General Practice

initiated a programme to devise guidelines for the provision of services. Criteria were written to determine access to publicly funded elective surgery. Treatment is given on the ability of patients to benefit (clinical and social), those with highest need would go first and those with little need may be refused.

The obvious disadvantage of either system is that the wealthy could by-pass it altogether and hence a two-tier system would, and has been, created. The poor do not have that option. Means testing may be an alternative to all care. Would a modest charge (say to see a GP) help? The answer is yes. Evidence shows this leads to a reduction in help-seeking behaviour. The alternative is to raise income tax. Hopefully evidence-based practice and guidelines from NICE will help avoid implicit rationing.

The Future of General Practice

PRIMARY CARE GROUPS

- PCGs were established throughout England in 1999
- Serve a population of about 100,000
- Accountable to Health Authority
- Resourced out of current fundholding allowances
- Involve all GPs and community nurses
- Primary Care budget to be fully cash limited
- Services commissioned by Primary Care Groups must meet national standards to ensure fair access and uniform quality
- PC Trusts to be managed by a Trust Board comprising GPs, nurses, managers, social services, representatives and lay people
- PCGs will eventually purchase 90% of hospital and community care
- As they show their ability to manage their budgets and services, they take increased responsibility by becoming free-standing primary care trusts
- Health Authorities will monitor standards, allocate resources, control progress to (or from) complete autonomy

Four grades with increasing independence
1. Provide advice on commissioning to Health Authority
2. Manage devolved budget
3. Independent Primary Care Trusts responsible for some commissioning
4. Independent Primary Care Trusts responsible for commissioning all primary and secondary care, with a fully integrated budget

Concerns
- Is there enough public health/management/commissioning expertise to support 500 PCGs?
- Will they be big enough/powerful enough to effect more than minor changes and improvements by providers?
- Will PCGs or Whitehall have ultimate control with regard to priorities, quality and equity?
- Will Health Authorities have the power of veto?
- Will devolving health care rationing to PCGs render them liable to litigation?
- What happens if they run out of money?
- Will devolving budgetary control to PCGs merely be a smokescreen to conceal NHS under funding?

160

The Future of General Practice

PERSONAL MEDICAL SERVICES (PMS) PILOTS

As a result of NHS (Primary Care) Act 1997, PMS schemes were designed to allow experimental schemes to test alternative models for delivering primary and community care.

British General Practitioners have traditionally been self-employed, the contract under which they perform work for the NHS is elaborate and is perceived as being inflexible and bureaucratic. This is termed General Medical Services (GMS), arrangements of which are set out in the 'Red Book'.

Although the Personal Medical Services scheme has sometimes been called the 'salaried doctors' scheme (to contrast with the normal self employment arrangements), this has not been its defining characteristic. The personal medical services scheme has been well received and a third wave of successful applicants is due to be announced towards the end of this year. There are several reasons for its popularity, although more recently it has been less popular.

- The scheme has generally succeeded in giving those taking part a perception of self determination and relative freedom from the constraints of NHS bureaucracy
- How much this perception is based on the active attitudes of the Health Authorities who hold the personal medical services contracts, and how much on the fact that these authorities have often not had the capacity to manage the scheme at all remains a moot point. Schemes in deprived areas were more likely to attract extra resources that were not generally available to practices working under the old regime, since GMS allocations are not usually linked to population needs.
- These resources have been used to create new services, liberate practitioners for professional development and improve facilities, especially for disadvantaged groups such as homeless and mentally ill people.

Aims
- Attract GPs to areas with recruitment problems
- Get GPs and community nurses to work more closely together
- Tackle inequalities and health problems of deprivation

The Future of General Practice

Different models for PMS exist:
- Salaried GP and nurse providing primary care to homeless
- Partnership of GP and nurse with joint responsibility for running a single practice
- Nurse Practitioners act as team leaders in a practice and/or employ their own salaried GPs
- Local practice to run a cottage hospital as a primary care and minor injuries unit
- NHS trust to employ salaried GPs to provide primary care under same roof as other community health services

Significance and implications
- All have an individual contract negotiated directly with their Health Authority, dispensing with the 'Red Book' and all its restrictions and limitations
- Break the monopoly of the single national contract
- Allow GPs to switch to salaried status, pass management responsibilities to others and concentrate on clinical work
- Give Primary Care Groups and Trusts a new tool for discharging their local responsibilities to provide primary care
- Offer great potential for innovation and service development
- Contractually obliged to deliver NSF guidelines in most cases

The Future of General Practice

OUT OF HOURS CARE AND 24 HOUR RESPONSIBILITY

Risks of split contract (day and night)
- Rolling, renewable contract could result in insecurity
- Other primary care providers may bid for out-of-hours work (e.g. Community Trusts, A&E Departments and BUPA)
- Further threatens integrity of GPs role, already at risk from hospital outreach, community paediatricians, community psychiatric teams, midwives etc.
- Dilution and fragmentation of GPs work
- Loss of control of care outside hospitals

Advantages	Disadvantages
<ul><li>Satisfaction from personal service</li><li>Educational benefits</li><li>Financial reward</li><li>Prevention of erosion of GPs role by other providers</li></ul>	<ul><li>Heavy workload – demand increased five-fold in last 25 years, two-fold in last three years</li><li>Stress may result in impaired quality of care at the time and impaired quality of care, the next day – burn out</li><li>Risk of violence</li></ul>

Deputising services
- Surveys show high degree of patient satisfaction
- Quality must be maintained
- Deputies must be well paid and well supported

1995 SETTLEMENT

1. GPs to keep 24 hour responsibility but can delegate more liberally
2. Fixed sum to be paid to each principal for out-of-hours cover
3. Same night visit fee for small rotas, large rotas and deputising service
4. Terms of service to be amended:
    - Allow wider range of out-of-hours services
    - Doctor can decide on
        - Advice only
        - Go to Primary Care Emergency Centre
        - House call

163

The Future of General Practice

- Deputies to be trained GPs registered with Health Authority, but need not be principals
- Deputies to be responsible for own actions

5. Primary Care Emergency Centres (PCECs) ?Where
   ?Staffed by GPs
   ?Open access or doctor referral only
   ?Funding

6. GPs able to apply for funds from Health Authority for:
   - Buying communication equipment
   - Developing PCECs for out-of-hours use
   - Defraying costs of arranging rotas
   - Locums in isolated rural areas
   - Using commercial deputising services

7. Educate patients: 'Be nice - think twice.'

The Future of General Practice

NHS DIRECT

Nurse-led 24 hour telephone helpline, available throughout England by the end of 2000.

Announced in December 1997 following the recommendations in the CMO's report *Developing Emergency Services in the Community*.
New service was to provide 'easier and faster advice and information for people about health, illness and the NHS so that they are better able to care for themselves and their families'.

CMO expressed the hope that a national telephone helpline might 'help reduce or limit the demand' on other parts of the NHS, in particular ambulance services, A&E departments and GP co-operatives.

In response to
- Growth of the 24 hour society
- Increasing demand for primary and emergency care
- Problems in recruiting and retaining nurses and GPs

Aims
- Reduce workload
- Provide easy access to an appropriate level of expertise
- Will empower patients with knowledge and thus foster self care

Long-term aims
- Health promotion, information centres, health guides, internet services

Concerns
- It will uncover unmet demand fuelling workload
- Will threaten continuity of care
- Telephone contact by nurses rather than a consultation with a GP may mean that important diagnoses are missed
- It will not be integrated with the rest of gateway services such as GP co-operatives
- Could result in waste of resources and patient confusion

Criticisms
- Service needs to be equally accessible to those without English as a first language, mentally ill people and elderly – they are less likely to use a telephone service

- Money for NHS Direct was not offered to existing primary care services to update the existing service arrangements
- Not enough liaison with GPs
- Lack of consistent advice in clinically identical cases

PAPERS:

 Evaluation of NHS Direct first wave sites, First interim report to the Department of Health
(Munro, 1998.)

Looked at three aspects of the service in the first three pilot sites:
- Descriptive account of the organisation and users of NHS Direct
- Caller satisfaction
- 'Before and after' assessment of its effects on other services

Showed that in the first 8 months:
- Demand was only one-third of that expected (expected to rise)
- Essentially used as an out-of-hours service with 72% of calls being out-of-hours
- Demographics reflected patterns for GP services, except that the elderly were under-represented
- Caller satisfaction rates were high
- Significant differences in the percentage of callers advised to attend A&E and/or their GP between three sites
- Significantly different advice given to 120 dummy cases (clinically identical) between three sites

A follow-up study by Munro *(BMJ 2000;321:150–3)* showed:
Same three pilot sites were studied over 24 months, in summary:
- No significant changes in uses of ambulance services and A&E Departments
- Changes in use of GP out-of-hours co-ops were small but significant (increase of 2% per month to a decrease of 0.8%)
- May have restrained increasing demand
- Overall, in the first year did not reduce or increase pressure on the NHS
- No evidence that it had uncovered extra demand
- Apparently is still popular with the public
- 'If NHS Direct has provided easier and faster advice and information and has improved access to health care for those who need it, then the fact that this has been achieved without

The Future of General Practice

increasing demand on other services seems encouraging'

WALK-IN CENTRES

Aims
- Offer people the opportunity to see a health care professional face to face on a walk-in basis
- Open from 7 am to 10 pm weekdays and weekends to provide information and treatment for minor conditions
- With or without appointments
- Centres will be funded initially for 3 years
- Same concerns that have been voiced regarding NHS Direct have been discussed with regard to walk-in centres
- Run by PCGs, Co-operatives, GPs and NHS Trusts

Objections
- Diversion of funds from other parts of primary care
- May generate additional demands
- Causes fragmentation of primary care and erosion of family doctor service which has:
  - Comprehensive medical record
  - Continuity of care at its core
  - Gatekeeper role

Benefits
- May reduce workload of GPs
- Responds to demand for wider access
- NHS Direct may help public make more appropriate use of health and social services.

The Future of General Practice

NURSE PRACTITIONERS

What work might they do?
- Prevention, immunisation, smears, contraception, review, BP, asthma, diabetes etc.
- Medical triage, independent management of minor illness with limited prescribing rights, referring to GP only when necessary
- Social triage – guiding patients needing social or financial help

How would GPs benefit?
- Over trained for much of what they do – less time on less complicated issues would mean more time for patients with more serious problems
- Skills learnt in training need no longer atrophy through disuse
- Potential for GPs to specialise in aspects of primary care
- Increased job satisfaction
- Improved morale
- Increased income through larger lists (e.g. 4,000 patients per doctor)

What are the possible problems?
- Dilution of continuity of care and of personal care
- GPs may feel themselves redundant
- Nurses may fail to diagnose rare but life-threatening conditions, or to spot unusual presentations
- More specialisation by GPs may lead to loss of 'generalist role'
- Cost of training programmes and salaries to be borne by Health Authorities
- Legal responsibility – nurses are responsible for own actions but GPs still have 'vicarious liability'
- Need to protect themselves by writing evidence-based protocols for delegated tasks
- Patients must be informed that they are not seeing a doctor so that they don't consent to procedures believing a doctor – not a nurse – will do them

What do the studies show?
They are:
- Safe
- Effective
- Popular with patients
- Good at listening, understanding and explaining

The Future of General Practice

- Good at following protocols
- Good at using drug formularies
- Less likely to prescribe
- More likely to use non-prescription
- Likely to advise on prevention approaches

How can they act as point of first contact?
- Triage
- Telephone advice
- Same day appointments
- Home visits

Effect on GPs
GPs report
- Reduced workload
- Increased satisfaction
- Improved standards of care
- More patients seen

What are the pitfalls? (This is food for thought not necessarily our views)
- 'Nurse Practitioner' title not regulated, the courses they go on are not externally assessed or regulated
- Are we in fact allowing non-medically-trained people to practise as doctors?
- Having to access a GP only via a nurse, is it acceptable that patients do not have a choice to see a doctor first?
- Introduction of a two-tier service with nurses providing much of the care in areas where it is difficult to recruit GPs, whereas leafy suburbs where GPs want to work are well staffed but patients have the least need – is this equitable?
- What effect would it have on the nature of General Practice?
- Ability to distinguish self-limiting from serious disease and the opportunity to develop a close rapport with patients are key skills of General Practitioners, would these be compromised?

What does a practice need before appointing a Nurse Practitioner?
- Job description to clarify role, responsibilities, accountability and liability
- Protocols and guidelines
- Formulary
- Education of staff on role of Nurse Practitioner
- Education of patients on role of Nurse Practitioner

What will the Nurse Practitioner need?
- Mechanisms of support/supervision/professional development, i.e. a mentor
- Mechanisms of problem resolution
- Training in protected time
- Accreditation scheme in addition to the Nurse Practitioner Degree
- Education funded by Health Authority
- Fewer prescribing restrictions

A themed issue of the BMJ *(2000;320:7241)* explored the changing roles of nurses in the NHS. Four trials of nurse impact on primary care were published.

 Nurse management of patients with minor illnesses in General Practice: a multicentre, Randomised Controlled Trial, Schum.
(BMJ 2000;320:1038)
Practice nurses attended a degree level course on managing minor illness for half a day for 3 months, also observed GPs in surgeries twice a week. Two month pilot period after the nurses were recruited. Patients asking for same day appointments with minor illness were randomly distributed between GP and Practice nurse.

Outcomes
- High satisfaction, both with doctor and nurse consultations (but significantly higher for nurses)
- Consultations with nurses took an average of 10 minutes and with doctors 8 minutes
- Similar prescription rates for a similar number of patients
- 73% of patients seen by nurses required no input from doctors
- Conclusion – practice nurses offer an effective service for people with minor illness

A further RCT study (Venning) in the same issue looked at cost effectiveness.

Showed that
- Nurse consultations were significantly longer than doctors' consultations
- They carried out more tests and asked patients to return more often
- There was no significant difference in patterns of prescribing or outcome

The Future of General Practice

- Patients were more satisfied with nurse consultations (allowing for time difference)
- No significant difference in health service costs between the two groups
- Conclusions were that costs were similar, but that if nurses could maintain the benefits whilst reducing their return consultation rates or shortening consultation times then they could be more cost effective than General Practitioners

The Future of General Practice

OUTREACH CLINICS

ADVANTAGES	DISADVANTAGES/CRITICISMS
• Improved communication between GP and consultant • Increased range of services in General Practice • Fewer people missing appointments • Reduced and more appropriate referral to hospital • Patient convenience • Better management • GP education	• Widens divide between progressive and inert practices • Inefficient use of consultant time • Inadequate facilities • No hospital records available • No diagnostic services available • Reduced consultant cover/teaching/research at hospital • Increased referral waiting time for patients of non-participating practices • Unnecessary referrals

The above are theoretical points as no evidence is available. As such, more evaluation is needed.

Q. *What are the costs to patient, GP and the hospital?*
Q. *How would they impact on referral, prescribing and effect on junior training (lack of consultant cover)?*

The Future of General Practice

PRACTICE FORMULARY

Aim
- Improved quality of care through rational, cost-effective prescribing

Criteria for inclusion
- Drugs must be necessary, safe, effective and economic

Method
- Develop own formulary
- Participate in development of district formulary
- Take over and amend established formulary

Benefits
- Education
- Generic prescribing increased
- Prescribing costs reduced
- Influence of drug companies reduced
- Prescribing policies/management policies agreed
- Self-audit
- Peer review

Problems
- Patients reluctant to change
- Doctors feel restricted
- Hospital initiate therapy with non-formulary drug

Q. How would you instigate a practice formulary?

The Future of General Practice

COMPUTER-GENERATED REPEAT PRESCRIPTIONS

The GMC have issued guidelines.
- Must take full account of your obligation to prescribe responsibly and safely
- Satisfy yourself it is safe to sign every repeat prescription
- Ensure provision is made for monitoring each patient's condition
- Ensure patients needing examination or assessment do not get repeat prescriptions without seeing a doctor, especially for drugs with potentially serious side-effects

Q. What is your responsibility for repeat prescriptions?

The Future of General Practice

POST-'SHIPMAN'

What are the long-term effects?
Alan Milburn ordered a wide-ranging enquiry into the issues raised by the case. The ramifications of which are still unknown as the death toll continues to grow.

GMC has been criticised for failing to hand over psychiatric reports on Shipman to the police; for allowing Shipman to return to practice after his drug conviction; for failing to inform West Pennine HA of Shipman's record and for failing to strike Shipman off the medical register immediately. Alan Milburn said the inquiry will lead to development of measures to safeguard against the risks of isolated medical practice.

Possible effects of the case on single handed/small practices
- *NHS plan* has given special consideration to small practices
- Additional requirements of revalidation
- Imposition of additional contractual quality requirements?
- Forced into PMS?
- However, repeated patient surveys show patient satisfaction is higher in single-handed practices than in group practices
- Also GPs can be professionally and individually isolated in group practices

An editorial in the BJGP by Mike Pringle (The Shipman Inquiry: Implications for the public's trust in doctors.*(BJGP 2000;50:454)*) looked at the implications of the Shipman case:
- Profession should be defending single-handed practices
- Professional isolation should be the focus
- Restore patient confidence by professional development, revalidation and appraisal
- Death certification will be investigated by the inquiry and it is likely that the second signatory on the cremation form will be a doctor who is appointed, trained and paid for the task, who will make appropriate enquiries into circumstances surrounding the death
- Death rates, although crude, may become part of any clinical governance monitoring system
- Stricter control of use and storage of controlled drugs

A somewhat stranger perspective on the whole tragic affair appeared in the next article. The author, a retired psychiatrist discussed serial homicide in the medical profession.

 Serial homicide by doctors: Shipman in perspective.
(Kinnell, BMJ 2000;321:1594–7)

Kinnell discussed that as a profession world-wide, doctors account for more notorious murderers than any other profession. He gives a historical perspective over the decades of other such cases in rather too much detail! Needless to say this will not be a 'Hot Topic' but we have included a snippet from the article. This is partly because we were surprised to find it was published at all, in such volatile times. For those of you who are interested please feel free to read the full article, otherwise we have quoted a few points.

- The previous BMA chairman, among others, is on record as saying that Harold Shipman is unique, yet medicine has arguably thrown up more serial killers than all the other professions put together
- Nursing comes a close second
- Dentistry too has had its notorious characters
- Among veterinarians homicide seems to be almost unknown
- The medical profession seems to attract some people with a pathological interest in the power of life and death
- Doctors have been responsible for killing not only patients and strangers but members of their own family
- The political killers par excellence were the Nazi doctors and the Japanese doctors engaged in biological warfare

CHAPTER 13: MEDICINE AND THE INTERNET

The Internet is transforming health care. It is creating a new conduit not only for communication but also in the access, sharing and exchange of information. Increasingly, patients are using the Internet to search for detailed information about their medical condition; they can obtain a second opinion from a 'cyberdoc' and can also check with various patient support groups about their best treatment options. The knowledge gained can then be used to challenge their doctor during subsequent consultations, which may then affect the doctor-patient relationship.

What makes the Internet attractive?
Doctors and other health care professionals want information as part of their everyday work. The Internet accelerates and broadens such provision. Patients often want more information and the Internet offers patients remedies.

It has been estimated that more than 25 million people use the Internet to search for health information. Medical information is thought to be one of the most retrieved types of information on the web. In fact, according to one survey, 27% of female and 15% of male Internet users access medical information regularly *(BMJ 1999;319:1294–6)*.

Through the Internet, patients not only have access to almost as much information as clinicians, but they are also starting to provide advice for other patients through websites that they host and manage. Even children can provide information for their peers, their parents and clinicians.

Is there any regulation of the information available on the Internet?
A major concern is the reliability of the information accessed, opinions offered, claims made and materials supplied by the Internet.

Health On the Net Foundation (www.hon.ch) is an international, non-profit making organisation based in Geneva. It provides a database of evaluated health materials and also promotes the use of the HON code as a self-governance initiative to help unify the quality of medical and health information available. Users of website health information displaying the HON logo can be assured that the material has been developed in accordance with these guidelines.

Medicine and the Internet

What problems may the Internet pose to health care professionals?
The biggest problem with obtaining health information from the Internet is that it is not always easy to decide what is reliable. As an example, one website has apparently reported the mortality for a certain type of bone cancer as 5%, while in reality it is closer to 75%! Estimates vary at the number of medically related sites are on the web, but they number at least 100,000. Only about **half** these sites have their content reviewed by doctors. In addition, many sites are American where the investigations and treatments for diseases is very different to those in UK which often causes confusion amongst patients.

Although data is not yet available, it is evident that clinicians can find themselves upstaged by and ill prepared to cope with patients who bring along information downloaded from the Internet.

More resources are needed to study the implications of the Internet for the role of patients and clinicians and also to ensure that the clinician-patient relationship is strengthened rather than undermined.

What is the NHS net?
By the end of 2000, all GP practices should have been connected to the NHS net. It has been proposed that Networked Electronic Health Records will be developed which will be available to all health care professionals 24 hours a day. All appointments and laboratory requests will be booked via the NHS net and community prescribing will also go electronic, with pharmacists accepting prescriptions via the Internet. An electronic library with health information for both the public and professionals will be available on the NHS net. The main concern of all this is confidentiality. It is, however, likely to take far longer to be running smoothly than the time proposed by the Government!

What are the problems with e-mail consultations?
The GPs Committee has recently produced a guide to online consulting (*'Consulting in the Modern World'*). This warns Practices that electronic communications systems could seriously damage the consultation process, may increase workload and also leave GPs open to legal action. It states that e-mail exchanges are best suited to arranging repeat prescriptions or booking appointments. In addition GPs are warned to always be wary of responding to patients who are abroad as this could potentially cause conflicts between overseas regulatory bodies and the General Medical Council.

178

Medicine and the Internet

SUMMARY POINTS ON MEDICINE AND THE INTERNET

- ❖ Medical information is very commonly searched for over the Internet
- ❖ Downloaded information is often very challenging to doctors
- ❖ Information is often inaccurate
- ❖ HON code is a self-governance initiative for health sites
- ❖ Confidentiality is still a concern

CHAPTER 14: ALTERNATIVE MEDICINE

Many more people are using alternative and complementary medicine; up to 10% of NHS physiotherapists currently use acupuncture. It has been estimated that alternative medicine is used by about 30% of the population in the UK, which is actually much less than Germany and USA. It is currently legal for anyone in the UK to practise alternative medicine without any training (except chiropracty and osteopathy).

The House of Lords select committee on Science and Technology recently recommended that in the interests of public safety the complementary medicine sector should be properly regulated and more research carried out into its effectiveness *(BMJ 2000;321:1365)*. Many complementary practitioners claim that their treatments are more cost-effective and safer than conventional medicine; however the evidence for this is still very scanty and weak.

Why is alternative medicine so popular?

Positive motivations	Negative motivations
• Perceived effectiveness and safety	• Dissatisfaction with (some aspect of) conventional care
• Control over treatment	• Poor doctor-patient relationship
• 'High touch, low tech'	• Insufficient time with doctor
• Pleasant therapeutic experience	• Long waiting lists
• Affluence	• Desperation
• Gives support in chronic illness – adds optimism to patients	

Herbal remedies

Why are herbal remedies so popular?
• False belief that natural plant products are harmless
• Conventional treatments are perceived as being ineffective or dangerous
• Trend towards ecological 'natural' living

With rationing looming in virtually all health care systems, the question of whether herbal medicines can save money is important. Not all herbal medicines are cheap. A standard daily dose of St John's Wort, for instance, will cost more than that of a tricyclic antidepressant.

What are some of the problems with herbal remedies?

There is a huge variation in the quality of different herbal medicinal preparations. Herbal remedies are sold as food supplements in the UK and so evade any regulation of their quality and safety.

- Some Chinese skin preparations contain aristolochic – a nephrotoxin
- A Chinese cold treatment contains a substance linked with liver toxicity and failure
- Some herbal medicines are deliberately contaminated with conventional medicines
- One herbal skin remedy for dermatitis was found to contain high doses of dexamethasone

What is St John's Wort?

St John's Wort (*Hypericum perforatum*) is an increasingly popular choice in the treatment of depression (see page 61) and there is plenty of evidence which shows that hypericum is as effective as imipramine in the treatment of mild to moderate depression *(BMJ 2000;321:536–9)*. In addition, the side-effects are fewer when compared with imipramine but as yet there have been no randomised controlled trials comparing SSRIs with St John's Wort. The use of St John's Wort is more limited than initially thought, as it is a liver inducer and therefore reduces levels of digoxin, carbamazepine, warfarin and the oral contraceptive pill. It has numerous interactions with other drugs, which patients should be warned of before starting it.

However, a recent randomised controlled trial involving 200 adults has actually shown St John's Wort is ineffective against major depression *(JAMA 2001;285:1978–86)*. This obviously highlights the need for further RCTs before St John's Wort can confidently be recommended for patients with depression.

What is ginkgo biloba?

A review of nine placebo-controlled, double-blind randomised trials of ginkgo biloba for dementia, covering 1497 patients, showed that ginkgo was more effective than placebo in delaying the clinical course of dementia (*Clin Drug Invest 1999;17:301–8*). It is, however, also a potent inhibitor of platelet activating factor so increases the risk of intracerebral haemorrhage in those people taking aspirin and warfarin.

Is there any good evidence available to support homeopathy?

There is currently insufficient evidence that homeopathy is clearly efficacious for any single clinical condition. For many of the conditions treated in homeopathic practice, such as depression, fatigue and eczema, randomised trials have not been undertaken. In addition, few of the existing studies of homeopathy have been independently replicated. However, many people have reported numerous benefits from homeopathy.

What are the implications to the doctor of patients receiving alternative therapy?

- Doctor may feel threatened or angry
- May need to review doctor-patient relationship
- May need to review consultation times and techniques
- Lack of information about patient's treatment from alternative practitioner
- Need to consider drug interactions with conventional medicine
- May even lead to misdiagnosis or mistreatment of patient

It is likely that complementary therapies will become more available on the NHS as further studies are done and the therapies evaluated properly.

 USEFUL WEBSITES

www.parliament.uk - full report from House of Lords select committee
www.medical-acupuncture.co.uk - British Medical Acupuncture Society
www.acupuncture.org.uk - British Acupuncture Council
www.bsmdh.org - British Society of Medical and Dental Hypnosis
www.osteopathy.org.uk - Osteopathic Information Service

SUMMARY POINTS FOR ALTERNATIVE MEDICINE

- ❖ 30% of UK population use alternative medicine
- ❖ Lack of good supportive RCTs
- ❖ Contents of herbal remedies vary widely
- ❖ Need to consider implications on doctor-patient relationship

CHAPTER 15: MEDICO-LEGAL ISSUES AND GUIDELINES

GENERAL MEDICAL COUNCIL (GMC)

The GMC licenses doctors to practise in the UK under the provisions of the Medical Act 1983. Its purpose is to make sure that the public are served by doctors who have the qualities it expects, and to protect the public from doctors whose conduct, professional performance or health places patients at risk.

What is 'Good Medical Practice'?
In 1995 the GMC published a comprehensive statement (or code) setting out the principles of *Good Medical Practice*, at the core of which it listed the *Duties of a Doctor* – which should be read carefully, for the exam as well as for good clinical practice! *Good Medical Practice* now sets the framework of professional standards within which doctors must practise within this country. Doctors accepting GMC registration are therefore making a commitment to their patients and to their profession to practise accordingly.

What are the 'duties of a doctor'?
Doctors as a profession have a duty to maintain a good standard of practice and care and also show respect for human life. The guidelines emphasise what is expected of a doctor in practice today; they state a doctor must, among other things:
- Make the patients their first concern
- Treat patients politely and considerately and respect their dignity and privacy
- Listen to patients and respect their views
- Give patients information in a way they can understand
- Respect the rights of patients to be fully involved in decisions about their care
- Keep their professional knowledge and skills up to date
- Recognise the limits of their professional competence
- Be honest and trustworthy
- Respect and protect confidential information
- Make sure their personal beliefs do not prejudice their patient's care
- Act quickly to protect patients from risk if they have good reason to believe they or a colleague may not be fit to practice
- Avoid abusing their position as a doctor
- Work with colleagues in the ways that best serve patients' interests

 USEFUL WEBSITE

www.gmc-uk.org – General Medical Council

Medico-legal issues and guidelines

COMPLAINTS

Complaints are a fact of life; the best approach is to manage them quickly and efficiently. Failure to satisfy a complainant at an early stage often results in entrenchment of positions and ultimately demands a much greater investment of time in resolving the conflict.

What are common complaints in primary care?
The majority of complaints in primary care are dealt with promptly and efficiently with minimal repercussions.

Common complaints include
- Complications of requests for visits
- Prescribing errors
- Delay or missed diagnosis
- Delay in referral
- Failure to explain investigation or treatment plans
- Breach of confidentiality
- Failure to seek consent
- Unacceptable attitude on the part of professionals

What is the complaints procedure?
The new NHS patient complaints procedure was introduced in April 1996 and has certain key objectives:
- Ease of access for patients and complainants
- A thorough and local resolution phase
- Fairness for both complainants and staff
- Investigation of complaints entirely separately from any subsequent disciplinary proceedings

The process for dealing with complaints is relatively simple
- The first stage is local resolution, to resolve the issue within the practice
- The second stage is an independent review
- The third stage is review by the Health Service Commissioner (Ombudsman) if requested by either the complainant or the doctor

How are complaints dealt with in primary care?
All GPs are now required under the terms of service to operate a practice-based complaints procedure. A complaints manager should be appointed within each practice (usually the practice manager).

184

Medico-legal issues and guidelines

The in-house procedure must be:
- Practice-owned and supported by all staff
- Adequately publicised with detailed written information

All complaints must
- Be dealt with at the time if a verbal complaint
- Be acknowledged within two working days
- Have a full written response and explanation within ten working days

Complainants should always be invited to discuss the matter with an attempt to resolve it at an early stage.

Medico-legal issues and guidelines

CONFIDENTIALITY

Confidentiality is the cornerstone of medical practice. Practitioners have a professional obligation to protect confidentiality and the presumption should always be made that **all** information is confidential. It is only under extreme circumstances (e.g. legal or moral duty) that confidentiality can be breached.

When can doctors disclose information without consent?
This question often crops up in the oral examination.

Disclosure of personal information without consent should **only** occur in the most exceptional circumstances; it may be justified when failure to do so may expose the patient or others to a risk of death or serious harm. Consent should be sought prior to disclosure where third parties are exposed to a risk so serious that it outweighs the patient's privacy interest. However, if this is not practicable, the information should be disclosed promptly to an appropriate person or authority.

This can occur in the following circumstances:
- Patient with an illness that is placing others at substantial risk (e.g. HIV)
- Patients continuing to drive against medical advice (see later)
- Where disclosure may assist in prevention, detection or prosecution of a serious crime
- Death certificates
- Statutory requirement (e.g. notification of communicable diseases)
- Following an order by a judge or presiding officer of a court
- When the patient is unable to give consent and it is in the patient's best interests (e.g. to relatives).

The GMC clearly states: *'Doctors who decide to disclose confidential information **must** be prepared to explain and justify their decision.'*

Under which circumstances can doctors disclose information to the DVLA?
The DVLA is legally responsible for deciding if a person if medically unfit to drive and patients have a legal duty to inform the DVLA of their medical condition if it affects their ability to drive. The patient's doctor must ensure that the patient understands that their medical condition may impair their ability to drive.

186

Medico-legal issues and guidelines

If patients are incapable of understanding the advice (e.g. dementia) the DVLA must be informed immediately.

If a patient refuses to inform the DVLA the doctor should make every reasonable effort to persuade the person to stop driving, which may even include telling the next of kin. If the patient cannot be persuaded to stop driving, the doctor should then disclose the relevant medical information immediately, in confidence, to the medical advisor of the DVLA. Before giving the information to the DVLA, the patient should be informed of the doctor's decision to do so. Once the DVLA has been informed, a letter should be written to the patient confirming that the disclosure has been made.

What is the Data Protection Act 1998?
This came into force in March 2000 and has significant implications for all health care professionals and it is important to be aware of the main provisions of this Act.

The Act means that
- Patients are entitled to see all manual and computer medical records
- All health records are now disclosable (previous deadline of 1 November 1991 under the Access to Health Records Act no longer applies)
- Application to do this should be made by written request
- Applicants can inspect his/her own record or request a readable copy
- The data must be disclosed within 40 days of receipt of the request
- A data controller can exclude information which breaches the confidentiality of, or relates to a third party who has not consented to disclosure
- Disclosure may be withheld if it were likely to 'cause serious harm to the physical or mental health or condition of the subject or any other person'

☐ SUMMARY POINTS FOR CONFIDENTIALITY

- ❖ Confidentiality must always be respected
- ❖ Should only be breached in extreme circumstances
- ❖ Data Protection Act has many implications

Medico-legal issues and guidelines

CONSENT

Most doctors are aware of the importance of obtaining consent from their patients but many are uncertain about what consent actually means and also fear that their instincts about what is right may not be enough to protect them from a legal challenge.

Any competent adult has the right to give or withhold consent to examination, investigation or treatment. Consent may be implied, oral or written. Consent should be based on information patients want to know and ought to know about their condition and treatment. This information should include:
- Details of the diagnosis and prognosis
- Results of undergoing treatment or refusing treatment
- Risks of uncertainties of treatment
- Possible complications of treatment

Patients may change their mind and withdraw their consent at any time. It should also be noted that no one can give consent for another adult; this is often not realised by many health care professionals.

What is meant by a 'competent adult'?
A competent adult must be able to
- Understand the nature and purpose of treatment
- Understand the benefits, risks and alternatives
- Understand the consequences of refusal
- Retain the information long enough to make an effective decision
- Make a free choice

Any mentally competent adult can refuse treatment for any reason (rational or irrational) or for **no** reason at all even if doing so may result in his or her own death. In addition, a competent pregnant woman may refuse any treatment, even if it would be detrimental to the fetus.

What about consent for incompetent adults?
For an incompetent adult the doctor should:
- Act in the patient's best interests
- Attempt to ascertain the patient's past wishes
- Review the medical and social knowledge of the patient's background, culture and religion
- Consult relatives, friends and carers
- Consider the option which least restricts the patient's future choices

188

Medico-legal issues and guidelines

Can children give their own consent?
Young people aged 16 and 17 are presumed to have the competence to give consent for themselves. Children under 16 years may give their consent if they are mature enough to understand the nature, purpose and possible consequences, risks and benefits of their decision and are not making the decision under duress. This is sometimes described as being 'Gillick competent'. Ideally the parents will be involved. If a competent child consents to treatment, a parent **cannot** override that consent. Legally, a parent can consent if a competent child refuses, but it is likely that taking such a serious step will be rare.

Failure to obtain a suitable consent may open a doctor to a GMC complaint, a civil claim or even criminal charges.

Case law on consent has evolved significantly over the past decade and the Department of Health has recently published an important and exceptionally useful guide on English law concerning consent for examination or treatment (see DoH website). A recent important development is the Human Rights Act 1998 which came into force in October 2000.

 USEFUL WEBSITES

www.dvla.gov.uk – Driving Vehicle Licensing Authority (Medical standard of fitness to drive)
www.gmc-uk.org- GMC website
www.doctor.stpaul.co.uk - The St. Paul website
www.doh.gov.uk/consent - Reference Guide to Consent for Examination or Treatment, Department of Health

---

SUMMARY POINTS FOR CONSENT

- ❖ Valid consent must always be obtained
- ❖ Competent adults can change their mind about consent
- ❖ Children are able to give their consent

Medico-legal issues and guidelines

MEDICAL NEGLIGENCE

It is widely known that the tide of medical litigation continues to rise. The MDU's recent figures indicate that there is an annual increase in litigation of 15%.

To pursue a medical negligence claim a patient has to prove, on the balance of probability (i.e. meaning more likely than not) three things:
- The doctor owed a duty of care
- There was a breach of that duty
- Harm followed as a result

What is the Bolam standard?
Independent medical doctors use the 'Bolam' standard to assess the doctor's clinical management. This means that the doctor has acted in a way that would be in agreement with a responsible body of doctors practising in the same field, and does not have to be the standard of the majority.

However, in cases such as Bolitho and Pearce, the courts have said that they will depart from the professional practice approach if they see fit, the ultimate tests being what the court thinks was a reasonable amount of information to give to the patient. This obviously leaves an element of doubt, as doctors cannot guess what the courts are going to say.

What is the commonest reason for a medical negligence claim?
A recent review of all claims involving GPs by the MDU found that almost half (45.5%) of all settled claims were related to a delay in a patient's diagnosis. A delay in diagnosis *per se* is not necessarily negligent, provided that the clinical management can be shown to be competent and reasonable.

However, the main problems are usually
- Failure to examine properly
- Inadequate follow-up arrangements
- Lack of appropriate investigations
- Reports misfiled in the notes
- Poor communication with colleagues and patients
- Poor medical record keeping

Medico-legal issues and guidelines

The increase in litigation in the UK does not reflect changing standards of clinical practice, which remain very high, but rather an increase in patient's expectations and their tendency to resort to litigation. The majority of claims do not go beyond disclosure of medical records and less than 5% get as far as a court hearing.

SUMMARY POINTS FOR NEGLIGENCE

- ❖ Bolam standard often still used
- ❖ Most claims are due to delayed diagnosis
- ❖ Harm must result for a negligence claim

Medico-legal issues and guidelines

GUIDELINES

Clinical guidelines have increasingly become a familiar part of clinical practice. They have been defined as 'systematically developed statements to assist practitioner and patient decisions about appropriate health care for specific clinical circumstances.' The BMJ has written a series of four articles on issues in the development and use of clinical guidelines *(BMJ 1999;318:527–30, 593–6, 661–4, 728–30)*. Clinical guidelines are only one option for improving the quality of care. They do, however, have both potential risks and harms.

Guidelines should be practical, realistic and based on valid up-to-date evidence. They should also be easily accessible to practitioners and should ideally be adapted to suit the local target population. They should always be practical and take into consideration the available resources needed for them to be successfully implemented. A poor example of this is the BTS guidelines for COAD where routine spirometry is recommended.

The successful introduction of guidelines is dependent on many factors including their clinical context and the methods used for developing, disseminating and implementing them. A recent survey revealed that although 45% of GPs have seen the National Osteoporosis Guidelines, only 22% had ever used them in their clinical practice *(Osteoporosis Review 1999; 7.2:1–3)*. This reflects the major difference between dissemination and implementation of guideline recommendation.

What are the benefits of guidelines?
- Improve consistency of care
- Empower patients to make more informed choices
- Improve quality of clinical decisions
- Can improve efficacy (save money)
- Reduce inappropriate practice

What are the problems with guidelines?
- Recommendations may be wrong
- May be biased
- May be inflexible and not relate to individual patient
- Evidence used to write the guidelines is not always from appropriate, well designed studies
- Can be time-consuming to use
- Need to be updated regularly
- Do not address all the uncertainties of clinical practice

Medico-legal issues and guidelines

What is the role of guidelines in court?
Guidelines could be introduced to a court by an expert witness as evidence of accepted and customary standards of care, but they cannot be introduced as a substitute for expert testimony. Courts are unlikely to adopt standards of care advocated in clinical guidelines as legal 'gold standards' because the mere fact that a guideline exists does not in itself establish that compliance with it is reasonable in the circumstances, or that non-compliance is negligent.

How easy is it to comply with guidelines?
A recent study in the BJGP has highlighted that it is not always easy to comply with guidelines, even if they are well-accepted. It showed that GPs targeted their actions regarding treatment for their patients with hypertension at diastolic BP of 100 mmHg rather than the recommended guideline of 90 mmHg, despite being aware of the guidelines *(BJGP 2001; 51:9–14)*.

Difficulties with always adhering to guidelines can be appreciated when considering the following clinical scenario:

A 68-year-old Type 2 diabetic patient presents at the end of a busy Friday afternoon surgery with a sore throat. You notice her blood pressure has not been taken for the past two years. You take it and find her BP to be 146/92! There are probably certain questions you might ask yourself when faced with a similar patient –
- What shall I tell the patient about their blood pressure?
- Is it likely that this patient's BP is consistently raised?
- Shall I arrange for her blood tests/ECG?
- Shall I start medication now with all its potential risks/side-effects?
- How will she react to taking another medication when she is already taking other regular medication?
- Will this patient realistically respond to advice re weight loss / lifestyle / smoking when she never has before?
- What is their compliance with medication really like?

Although you know the BTS guidelines it is not always that easy to stick to them!

Guidelines are essentially written for the management of patient populations rather than for individuals. They will not address all the uncertainties of current clinical practice and should be seen as only one strategy that can help improve the quality of care that patients receive. Although guidelines are meant to tackle variations in practice there is

Medico-legal issues and guidelines

always a risk of standardising practice around the average, which is not necessarily always the best for every clinical situation *(BMJ 1993;43:146–51)*.

☐ **SUMMARY POINTS FOR GUIDELINES**

❖ Only one option for improving care
❖ Should ideally suit the local target population
❖ Numerous benefits and drawbacks
❖ Do not address all the uncertainties of clinical practice

CHAPTER 16: ADVANCE DIRECTIVES

An advance directive is a document by which a person can state, in advance of becoming incompetent, that he or she wishes to authorise or refuse certain forms of medical treatment.

- Now legally binding on doctors in common law High Court 1994 (however no formal legislation at present). Law Commission has proposed legislation to put Advance Directives on a statutory basis (1995).
- Endorsed by UK medical and legal professions
- BMA code of practice issued April 1995
- From October 1999, people in England and Wales have been able to appoint a friend or relative to take health care decisions if they lose the ability to make their own decisions
- Drawn up when patient has full mental capacity, the 'Continuing Power of Attorney' allows the 'proxy decision maker' to take healthcare, welfare and financial decisions
- The Court of Protection can, if necessary, appoint a manager (relative, social worker) to handle incapacitated persons' affairs

An Advanced Directive should
- Be made by people who are competent to do so, be able to understand, retain and act on the information on which the refusal to treat is based
- Be presumed to be valid if signed and witnessed
- Be revocable if the patients are competent to revoke it
- Explicitly state the author's awareness that death might or will be the result of the directive
- Not preclude the provision of basic care, defined as the maintenance of bodily cleanliness, relief of sustained pain and the provision of oral nutrition and hydration
- NOT be deliberately ignored, such action being a criminal offence

Other considerations
Competence is best confirmed by having a person's signature witnessed by two people, one of whom should be a doctor capable of attesting to the person's state of mind.

Advance Directives

END OF LIFE DECISIONS

- The Dutch have done most of the work in this field
- Doctors make end of life decisions in about 40% of deaths in the UK
- 75% involve withdrawal or withholding of treatment
- Doses of opiates likely to end life in 25%

'Withholding and withdrawing life-prolonging treatment' – Guidelines by BMA 1999

The key principles are
- Life cannot be preserved at all costs – treatment must be more of a benefit than a burden
- Artificial nutrition and hydration constitutes medical treatment
- Competent patients have the legal right to refuse treatment
- Where patients cannot express their view, doctors must take account of previously expressed wishes, the likelihood of any improvement and the likelihood of the patient experiencing severe pain or suffering
- Close co-operation with the other professionals in the team is vital in decision-making
- All proposals to withdraw or withhold artificial nutrition and hydration should be formally reviewed by a senior clinician who is not part of the team

'Doctrine of double effect'

States that if measures taken to relieve physical or mental suffering cause the death of a patient, then it is morally and legally acceptable provided the doctor's intent is to relieve distress and not to kill the patient.

In general the doctor must make a full assessment of the patient's condition, consult with relatives, carers and other healthcare professions involved in the case and ask for a second medical opinion either from a specialist or from another GP.

PAPERS:

 Physician assisted suicide, euthanasia or withdrawal of treatment.
Churchill.
(BMJ 1997;315:137–8)

The Oregon Death with Dignity Act was passed in 1994. It allows primary care physicians to comply with a request for lethal drugs from a competent patient with less than six months to live.

Holland has become the testing ground for the world, although assisting with requested euthanasia remains a criminal act, Dutch doctors have not been prosecuted when they follow strict guidelines.

Recent Editorials in BMJ

 Do not resuscitate (DNR) decisions
In 2000 the British Medical Association, the Resuscitation Council (UK) and the Royal College of Nursing jointly said that DNR orders could be considered only after discussion with the patient or others close to the patient. Age Concern's dossier is evidence that this guideline is being flouted (they have 50 case histories of inappropriate DNR decisions).

Resuscitation after a cardiopulmonary arrest is effective in only one in five patients. Although it may be appropriate to withhold resuscitation when a patient is dying, failure to involve patients in decisions on DNR orders negates their autonomy. It is most unfair for age to be used as a criterion to withhold cardiopulmonary resuscitation. Most patients and relatives consider that discussions about death and DNR orders are essential aspects of planning their care. It is doctors and nurses who find such discussions painful.

DNR orders are increasingly used and have greater implications than merely not calling the resuscitation team. Over two-thirds of patients with DNR orders are not involved in making these decisions. After adjustment for disease severity, prognostic factors, age and other co-variates, patients given these orders are more than 30 times more likely to die, suggesting that DNR orders may reduce quality of care. DNR orders are more commonly used in the USA for black people, alcohol misusers, non-English speakers and people infected with HIV, suggesting that doctors have stereotypes of those who are not worth saving.

Advance Directives

 The role of the court in decisions about medical treatment
- Circumstances occur in which it is necessary or wise to obtain authority from a court as to the lawfulness of proposed medical treatments when patients are not capable of consenting or have refused consent to such interventions
- In cases of permanent vegetative states, the court's authority must be obtained before artificial nutrition and hydration is withdrawn
- In other cases the courts can protect doctors from criticism and claims that they have acted unlawfully
- In the case of adults, the legal criteria are whether patients lack the capacity to give or refuse consent and if so what is in their best interests; in the case of children, welfare is the paramount consideration

 Dealing with children
- Those having parental responsibility, usually the parents, can give consent to medical treatment
- If the parents refuse consent to treatment recommended by the doctors, it will be necessary (and possible) for the consent to be supplied instead through an order of the court
- There is a starting point that the united view of both parents is correct in identifying where their child's welfare lies
- Cancelled out where the court finds on the evidence that their view is contrary to the welfare of the child
- It is well established that, for example, although Jehovah's Witnesses may in accordance with their religious beliefs withhold consent to blood transfusions for themselves as adults, if their children's lives are endangered the courts will provide the missing consent for the administration of blood
- When a child is able to express his or her own view, this becomes a factor in the decision about treatment. The courts have described a category of child as 'Gillick Competent' (of sufficient understanding and intelligence to understand fully the specific treatment proposed).
- A court may use its inherent jurisdiction to override the refusal of consent if satisfied that is what the welfare of the child requires

 The Special Position of 16–18 year olds
- Section 8 of the Family Law Reform Act 1969
- Able to give consent to medical treatment as if they were adult
- It does not, however, follow that if they refuse to give their consent

and are on the face of it capable of making that decision, their refusal will be determinative in the same way as it would be if they were adult
- No minor of any age has power, by refusing treatment, to override a consent given by the court or by a person having parental responsibility.
- The child's level of competence is relevant in assessing the weight to be given to his or her views, but these views will not determine the issue
- The paramount consideration is the welfare of the child

PAPERS:

 The separating of conjoined twins
(Smith, BMJ 2000;321:782)

- This controversial case of conjoined twins was recently decided by the Court of Appeal in England
- What is the legal significance of this case?
- The parents did not want Jodie to be saved at the cost of Mary's life. They took the view that this would be to end a life, a position in which their Catholic Church supported them. In these circumstances the first issue that the court had to address was whether parents could refuse to allow treatment.
- Here the court applied a well-established principle of English law, which is that judges can overrule parental opposition to treatment if it is in the best interest of the child to do so. This is the so-called 'welfare principle'.
- In a normal case that would have been enough, but this was no ordinary case. The judges were at pains to hold that Mary's life had intrinsic value, even if she was dependent on her sister and had no hope of a reasonable quality of life.
- Then there was the issue of 'criminal law'. The judges might decide to favour one child over another, but they could not authorise a procedure that could amount to homicide. At this point the principle of 'necessity' entered the courtroom.
- 'Necessity' is a broad criminal law defence, that may authorise an otherwise criminal act provided that the act is the lesser of two evils
- The judges have made it abundantly clear that the value of every human life must be upheld, and it is only when there is absolutely no alternative but to make a choice between lives that this will be

Advance Directives

permitted. This decision acknowledges that the making of a hard choice in favour of one life over another may be defensible in legal terms. Critics of this decision will say that it represents a further step towards the legal recognition of euthanasia. This is not so. What it does is to endorse the position that, although human life is of the greatest value, no good end is necessarily served by taking an absolutist position.

CHAPTER 17: MISCELLANEOUS TOPICS

REFUGEES

The issues regarding refugees, asylum seekers and immigration have all been visible in the media for the last few years. Whatever views you have on the subject, it is abundantly clear that that there are groups of people in our society who in most cases have been uprooted from their homes because of fear, famine and war. We have a responsibility to provide them with a quality health care service that we would afford our own population. Hypothetically, if the tables could be turned, we are fairly sure we would want the same. The refugee issue can provide a fruitful amount of ethical questions, especially when the health care element is introduced.

The issues of refugees was discussed in the summary below:

 Refugees and primary care: tackling the inequalities
(BMJ 1998;317:1444.)

This interesting article appeared in the BMJ when a large number of refugees were arriving in England from the troubles in the Balkans. As the 20th century draws to a close, outbreaks of hatred between human population groups show no sign of abating and conflicts continue to erupt. Families across the world find themselves forced to leave their homes and seek refuge where it can be found. Globally, there are 18 million refugees with 230,000 living in the UK. Almost half of these live in London, where 100,000 people are refugees or awaiting confirmation of refugee status. Many refugees have health problems but experience difficulty having their needs met by the NHS. This article explores the challenges that refugees pose for primary care and suggests alternative strategies to address inequalities in the care of refugees.

- The refugee population in Britain is highly diverse and is likely to remain large as conflicts continue to occur throughout the world
- Refugees, unlike other migrants, have had to flee to escape oppression
- The refugee population is concentrated in the greater London area, but new legislation will result in dispersal throughout the UK
- Refugees may be vulnerable to mental health problems yet have difficulty communicating their needs because of language barriers
- All refugees are entitled to the full range of NHS services free of charge, including registration with a General Practitioner

Miscellaneous Topics

- A strategic approach is needed to address the inequalities in primary care

Definition of refugees
- Those applying for asylum (refugee) status in the UK
- Those who have been given temporary admission by the immigration service while their applications are considered
- Those who have been given exceptional leave to remain in or enter the country
- Those who are required to renew their status at the Home Office at regular intervals
- Those given refugee status
- Those who gain the right to stay in this country indefinitely
- Those who have had their application refused and are going through the appeals process
- Dependants of the above groups
- Other individuals or groups who may fall outside the legal definition but who face similar problems: such as those entering the country under family reunion rules, policy or discretion

What happens to refugees?
- Refugee population is not evenly spread
- Concentrated in areas where local authorities have given refugee housing a higher priority
- Legislation will result in greater dispersal of refugees, which will make the provision of specialist services more difficult
- 'Cultural bereavement' and coping with 'deeply disruptive change' are widely shared experiences of migration
- Refugees are distinguished from other migrants by their lack of choice
- Refugees have had to leave their countries of origin to escape persecution, imprisonment, torture or even death
- Families may have been physically separated, causing much grief
- Refugees are often preoccupied by worry about relatives left behind in their country of origin
- Many refugees, including children, have no other relatives in the UK
- Poverty and dissatisfaction with housing is widespread

Health problems
- A recent UK study of Iraqi refugees found that all had been separated involuntarily from some close family members
- 65% had a history of systematic torture during detention

202

Miscellaneous Topics

- 29% were unable to speak any English
- Over 50% had significant psychological morbidity
- Evidence that refugees who have not yet been granted the right to remain are under particular stress

Deficiencies of primary care
- All refugees are entitled to the full range of NHS treatment free of charge
- All refugees have the right to register with a GP
- There is evidence that some GPs are confused about this
- Some patients are asked for passports when trying to register, which raises a number of questions:
  - What happens to patients unable to produce a valid passport?
    - Are they sent away?
    - Who makes these decisions?
- Some practices are, perhaps reluctantly, open for refugees whereas others are effectively closed, creating neighbouring practices with very different demographic profiles and unequal needs
- When refugees join a GP's list they are often registered on a temporary rather than a permanent basis
- This removes financial incentives to undertake immunisation and cervical smear tests

Why do General Practitioners avoid giving refugees permanent registration status?
- High mobility of refugees is a myth – 70% of refugees had been living in their current home for more than a year (Home Office Survey 1995)
- Language barriers at the reception desk and in the consultation are common
- Health authorities lack interpreter services, generally not available outside working hours
- Telephone interpreting using 'hands free' technology may offer a solution
- Lack of adequate professional interpreting services presents a barrier for all non-English speaking patients, but this barrier is larger for those with psychological and emotional difficulties

Q. If tragic mistakes are made as a result of communication failure does moral responsibility rest with the doctor or with a medical system which expects doctors to communicate well but fails to provide adequate resources?

Miscellaneous Topics

Increasing spending on refugee primary care
- Is fully justifiable on clinical and ethical grounds
- Recognise that it requires considerable political courage to prioritise refugees at a time when other groups in the population, such as elderly people and the mentally ill, have been identified as in need of greater resources
- It is important to remember that many refugees who settle in Britain have made valuable contributions to society

What can be done to improve primary care for refugees?
- A strategic approach is required
- Intensive courses in spoken English
- The DoH needs to commission an information pack that includes a certificate of entitlement to NHS treatment and to develop patient held medical records
- The development of a national telephone interpreting service in a range of languages is a priority
- A separate capitation payment for refugee patients, together with a new item of service payment linked to the duration of each professionally interpreted consultation, should be introduced
- Health care facilitators should be recruited from each specific refugee population and could help to provide patient held records with an accurate and detailed medical history and support health promotion and screening

Conclusion
- The refugee population is likely to remain large
- High needs, especially psychological distress, combined with language barriers require a great deal of additional time in consultations
- GPs in inner cities need adequate resources, especially interpreting services and should be properly rewarded
- A truly effective solution requires the political will to develop a comprehensive strategy at national level

Miscellaneous Topics

RECENT ETHICAL ADVANCES

 Clinical review – Recent advances in medical ethics.
(BMJ 2000;321:282)

This interesting review focused on the continuing evolution of medical ethics through new technology, some of which could be envisaged making good viva material.

Goal of medical ethics is to improve the quality of patient care by identifying, analysing and attempting to resolve the ethical problems that arise in practice.

Review advances in five areas:
1. End of life care
2. Medical error
3. Priority setting
4. Biotechnology
5. Medical ethics education
+ two future issues: 'eHealth' and 'global bioethics'

1. End of life care
See previous chapter.

2. Medical error
The main recent advance is the development of the Tavistock principles, which serve as an ethical foundation for those working to improve medical error.

All the Tavistock principles are relevant to the problem of medical error, but the most important are:
- Co-operation with each other and those served is the imperative for those working within the health care delivery system
- All individuals and groups involved in health care, whether providing access or services, have the continuing responsibility to help improve its quality
- In developing a culture of safety, clinicians will need to act as role models for their students by applying these principles themselves the next time they encounter a medical error
- Healthcare leaders will need to 'feel personally responsible for error' and 'declare error reduction to be an explicit organisational goal and [devote] a significant proportion of the board and management agenda…to achieving this goal'.

Miscellaneous Topics

3. Priority setting
Development of an ethics framework, 'Accountability for Reasonableness', for legitimate and fair decisions on setting priorities.
Priority setting = 'rationing' 20 years ago = 'resource allocation' 10 years ago and will be called 'sustainability' 10 years from now.

The four conditions of 'Accountability for Reasonableness'

- **Publicity**

Decisions regarding coverage for new technologies (and other limit setting decisions) and their rationales must be publicly accessible.

- **Relevance**

These rationales must rest on evidence, reasons and principles that fair-minded parties (managers, clinicians, patients and consumers in general) can agree are relevant to deciding how to meet the diverse needs of a covered population under necessary resource constraints.

- **Appeals**

There must be a mechanism for challenge and dispute resolution regarding limit setting decisions, including the opportunity for revising decisions in light of further evidence or arguments.

- **Enforcement**

There must be either voluntary or public regulation of the process to ensure that the first three conditions are met.

4. Biotechnology
- Emerging consensus on the acceptability of stem cell research
- The UK Nuffield Council on Bioethics has issued a report supporting stem cell research
- Latest in a series of important consensus documents on biotechnology such as the *'WHO's guiding principles on medical genetics and biotechnology'* and the *'Human Genome Organization's'* statement on benefit sharing
- Stem cells are 'cells with the capacity for unlimited or prolonged self-renewal that can produce at least one type of highly differentiated descendant'
- The clinical potential of stem cells is enormous, including neuronal repair, haematological reconstitution and organ transplantation
- The problem with embryonic stem cells is that they are derived from human embryos. Opponents of embryonic stem cell research

Miscellaneous Topics

are concerned with the moral and legal status of the embryo and advocate a moratorium.
- Proponents, however, focus on the potential benefits to patients
- Recent reports suggest that adult stem cells can differentiate into developmentally unrelated cell types - this would mitigate the ethical tensions related to embryonic stem cells

5. Medical ethics education
- The revolution in information technology will dramatically change medical practice
- Many ethical issues, including confidentiality of electronic medical records and the relation of clinical records to research and management of health systems
- Dramatic changes in the way doctors learn and access medical literature are in question

eHealth
- The revolution in information technology will dramatically change medical practice
- This raises many ethical issues, including how we can keep electronic medical records confidential and how we use our patient data to research and manage health systems.
- Doctors will also dramatically change the way they learn and access medical literature
- A code of ethics for 'eHealth' has been developed by the Internet Healthcare Coalition, an organisation with representatives from industry, academic groups, patient and consumer organisations

A draft of the code can be found at

 www.ihealthcoalition.org/ethics/draftcode.html

Global bioethics
- In this era of advanced globalisation the problems of medical ethics can no longer be viewed only from the perspective of wealthy countries.
- Global bioethics seeks to identify key ethical problems faced by the world's six billion inhabitants and envisages solutions that transcend national borders and cultures
- An International Association of Bioethics has been formed and a discussion board on global bioethics has been launched

CHAPTER 18: THE CONSULTATION

- All would agree that the consultation is central to our speciality
- Lack of time in consultations is the main criticism of GP services in patient surveys
- Consultations in the UK are generally shorter than in the rest of the developed world

Richardson *(JR Coll Gen Pract. 1973–Mar;23(128):155)* found that consultations with faster doctors contained all the components of consultations with slower doctors but that everything was done fractionally faster.

Howie *(Fam Pract. 1991 Sep;8(3):253–60)* found that longer consultations were associated with doctors dealing with more psycho-social problems, chronic health problems, health promotion and higher patient satisfaction.

Wilson and colleagues *(BMJ 1992;304(6821):227–30)* showed that increasing a consultation by an average of '1 minute' significantly increased the amount of health promotion given during the course of the consultation.

 Quality at General Practice consultations: cross sectional survey
(Howie, BMJ 1999;319:738–43)
Questionnaire study completed by 25,000 adults attending a randomly selected group of practices over two weeks. Looked at patient enablement, duration of consultation, familiarity with their doctor and size of the practice list.

Results showed
- Mean duration of consultations was 8 minutes
- Individual consultations enablement score was most closely linked with the duration of the consultation and knowing the doctor well
- Doctors from small practices enabled their patients more than those from large practices
- Concluded that it may be time to reward doctors with longer consultations and to promote continuity of care

Patients unvoiced agendas in General Practice consultations: qualitative study
(Barry, BMJ 2000;320:1246–50)
- 20 General Practices in South East England and the West Midlands
- 35 patients consulting 20 General Practitioners in appointment and emergency surgeries
- Questionnaire prior to the consultation to elicit patient agendas for the consultation
- Consultation was taped and the doctor interviewed about the consultation the next day
- Patients were re-interviewed one week later to discuss the outcome of the consultation

Results showed
- Patients have about 5 items on their agenda per consultation
- Usually a mixture of symptoms and psychosocial issues
- Voiced agenda items were most commonly:
  - Symptoms
  - Requests for diagnoses
  - Prescriptions
- Unvoiced agenda items were:
  - Worries about possible diagnosis
  - What the future holds
  - Patient's ideas about what is wrong, side-effects
  - Not wanting a prescription/information relating to social context
- Only 4/35 patients voiced their full agendas
- 24 patients voiced all their symptoms but social and emotional issues were more likely to remain unvoiced
- Both doctors and patients may not be open to the presentation of a fuller agenda, the doctors perhaps lacking in confidence and seeing them as overly time consuming. The patients worried about what is deemed appropriate to communicate and about wasting doctor's time
- More effective consultation leads to improved outcomes and by changing doctor's views and behaviours, patients may also be facilitated to change
- Active steps should be taken in daily practice to encourage voicing of patient's agendas

The Consultation

 Preferences of patients for patient centred approach to consultation in primary care: observational study
(Little, BMJ 2001;322:468)

Consecutive patients in the waiting room of three doctors' surgeries took part. One in a deprived area of a large provincial city, the second a training practice serving an urban population of a cathedral city and the third a training practice in a market town serving a mixed urban-rural population; characteristics of the sample were similar to the attending sample from the national morbidity survey.

- 865 patients participated: 95% returned the questionnaire and were similar in demographic characteristic to national samples
- Patients were given questionnaires prior to seeing the GP asking them to agree or disagree on questions about what they wanted the doctor to do in the consultation
- It focused on communication (agreed with by 88–99% of patients), partnership (77–87%) and health promotion (85–89%).
- Fewer wanted an examination (63%) and only a quarter wanted a prescription
- Patients who strongly wanted good communication were more likely to feel unwell, be high attenders and have no paid work
- Strongly wanting partnership was also related to feeling unwell, worrying about the problem, high attendance and no paid work
- Those strongly wanting health promotion and those worried about their problem were high attenders
- Patients who wanted a prescription were more likely to want good communication, partnership and health promotion
- Patients wanting a prescription were more likely to be unmarried, have a partner with no paid work, no education beyond GCSE and be aged over 60
- Those wanting an examination were more likely to have no education beyond GCSE and feel worried about their problem
- Patients required about 3–5 minutes to complete the questionnaire before seeing the doctor so those seeing doctors running on time (a small minority) could not be approached
- Time limitation meant fewer questions asked

The Consultation

Key points
- They concluded patients in primary care strongly want a patient-centred approach, with communication, partnership and health promotion
- Improved communication can improve satisfaction and biomedical outcomes
- Involving patients in partnership can have benefits without increasing their anxiety and with the potential to reduce side-effects of prescribing
- Patients with a very strong preference for patient-centredness are those who are vulnerable either socioeconomically or because they are feeling particularly unwell or worried

The Consultation

THE DOCTOR-PATIENT PARTNERSHIP

An entire edition of the BMJ was devoted to this issue on 18 September 1999.

📖 *Paternalism or Partnership*
Coulter (Editorial)

- Key to successful doctor-patient partnerships is to recognise that patients are experts too
- Doctors should be well informed about diagnostic techniques, the causes of disease, prognosis, treatment options and prevention strategies
- Only the patient knows about his experience of health or illness, social circumstances, habits and behaviour, attitudes to risk, values and preferences
- Both types of knowledge are needed to manage illness successfully so both parties should be prepared to share information and take decisions jointly
- The Government is promoting the patient partnership – it is encouraging self care through a new handbook of common ailments, availability of advice via the Internet and telephone advice help lines

Decision-making aids were also reviewed in this edition.
- Showed that they were better than usual care in improving patient's knowledge
- Comfort and participation in decision-making without increasing anxiety
- Had little effect on satisfaction and variable effect on patient's decisions

Another study looked at how to communicate risks versus benefit of interventions to patients:
- Concluded that a range of risk communication tools in different formats was helpful
- These involved verbal descriptions of risk, numerical data and graphical depiction, which was thought to be effective and saved time in the consultation

One study looked at the response of GP registrars to shared decision making with patients:
- Registrars reported not receiving training in the skills needed to successfully involve patients in decision making
- Training needs will have to be addressed if shared decision making is going to become a reality

212

The Consultation

CONSULTATION MODELS

BIOMEDICAL MODEL

The classic medical diagnostic process

• Observation	History and examination
• Hypothesis	Provisional diagnosis
• Hypothesis testing	Investigations
• Deduction	Definitive diagnosis

In essence is a *hypothetico-deductive* model but:

Reductionist:	Patient regarded as collection of signs, symptoms and diagnosis
Doctor centred:	Patient's ideas, concerns and expectations Sharing information Agreeing management plan

- No progress can be made if no objective physical disorder unearthed
- Omits use of doctor-patient relationship

ALTERNATIVE MODELS

- More holistic
- Not competing, but complementary
- Several are often needed to give broad understanding of something as complex as human interaction

TRIAXIAL MODEL

Address patient's problem in

- Physical terms
- Psychological terms
- Social terms

The Consultation

BYRNE AND LONG

Phase I — The doctor establishes a relationship with the patient.

Phase II — The doctor either attempts to discover or actually discovers the reason for the patient's attendance.

Phase III — The doctor conducts a verbal or physical examination or both.

Phase IV — The doctor, or the doctor and the patient, or the patient (in that order of probability) consider the condition.

Phase V — The doctor, and occasionally the patient, detail further treatment or further investigation.

Phase VI — The consultation is terminated, usually by the doctor.

Used the terms Doctor Centred and Patient Centred. This model was produced after analysing over 2,000 tape recordings of consultations.

STOTT AND DAVIS

Management of presenting problems	**Modification of help-seeking behaviour**
Management of continuing problems	**Opportunistic health promotion**

PENDLETON, SCHOFIELD, TATE AND HAVELOCK
SEVEN TASKS

1. To define the reason for the patients attendance, including:
   - The nature and history of the problems
   - Their aetiology
   - The patient's ideas, concerns and expectations
   - The effects of the problems.

2. To consider other problems:
   - Continuing problems
   - Risk factors

The Consultation

3. With the patient, to choose an appropriate action for each problem.

4. To achieve a shared understanding of the problems with the patient.

5. To involve the patient in the management and encourage him to accept responsibility.

6. To use time and resources appropriately:
  - In the consultation
  - In the long-term

7. To establish or maintain a relationship with the patient which helps to achieve the other tasks.

Emphasises the importance of the patient's view and understanding of the problem. Includes the term 'Consultation Mapping.'

NEIGHBOUR
THE INNER CONSULTATION

Connecting	Needs rapport building skills.
Summarising	Needs listening and eliciting skills to facilitate effective assessment.
Hand Over	Needs communicating skills to hand over responsibility for management.
Safety Netting	Needs predicting skills to suggest contingency plan for worst scenario.
House Keeping	Needs self-awareness to clear mind of psychological remains of one consultation so that it has no detrimental effect on the next.

ROSENSTOCK, BECKER AND MAIMAN
HEALTH BELIEFS MODEL

It shows that the patient is more likely to accept advice, diagnosis or treatment if the doctor is aware of their ideas, concerns and expectations.

The Consultation

Patient's behaviour is determined by:
- Alarming symptoms
- Trigger factors such as advice from family and friends, messages from media
- Health motivation (interest in health)
- Perceived vulnerability to the condition
- Perceived seriousness of the condition
- Perceived balance of benefits of treatment against costs
- Belief that doctor has/has not understood patient's concerns

HERON
SIX CATEGORY INTERVENTION MODEL

Doctor can use any of six types of intervention.

1. **Prescriptive**   Instructions
    Advice

2. **Informative**   Explanations
    Interpretations
    New knowledge

3. **Confronting**   Feedback on behaviour
    Challenging but caring attitude

4. **Cathartic**   Aiding release of emotions in form of anger, laughter, crying

5. **Catalytic**   Encouraging patient to explore feelings, thoughts and behaviour

6. **Supportive**   Bolstering self-worth

The Consultation

BERNE
TRANSACTIONAL ANALYSIS 'Games People Play'

- Explores behaviour within relationships
- Identifies three 'ego-states': Parent – critical or caring
                                  Adult – logical
                                  Child – spontaneous or dependent
- Examines implications of, and reasons for, the different states
- Explores 'games' – useful for analysing why consultations repeatedly go wrong and encouraging doctors to break out of these unproductive cycles of behaviour

BALINT
THE DOCTOR, HIS PATIENT AND THE ILLNESS (1957)

The Doctor-Patient Relationship is fundamental.
Patients are more than broken machines, and doctors have feelings, which have a function in the consultation. Proposed that:
- Psychological problems are often manifested physically and even physical disease has its own psychological consequences which need particular attention
- Doctors have feelings and those feelings have a function in the consultation
- There needs to be specific training to produce limited but considerable change in the doctor's personality so that they could become more sensitive to the patient's thoughts during the consultation.

The doctor must:
- Discover the patient's beliefs, concerns and expectations about the problem or problems presented
- Share their own understanding of the problems with the patient in terms that are understood by the patient
- Share the decision making with the patient
- Encourage the patient to take appropriate responsibility for their own health

The Consultation

Key concepts and phrases from Balint, are listed below. For the exam, it is helpful to think of consultations when they may occur.

1. The doctor as a drug

2. The child as the presenting complaint
- May offer another person (e.g. child) as the problem when there are underlying psycho-social problems

3. Elimination by appropriate physical examination
- Mistaken beliefs in the origin of symptoms are reinforced by examination
- May reinforce that neurotic symptoms are in fact due to physical illness

4. Collusion of anonymity
- Responsibility of uncovering underlying problems becomes increasingly diluted by repeated referral
- No one takes responsibility

5. The mutual investment company
- Formed and managed by the doctor and the patient
- 'Clinical illnesses' equal 'Offers' in a long relationship
- 'Offers' of problems (physical and psycho-social) are presented to the doctor for his 'Acceptance'

6. The flash
- When the real reason of the 'Offer' (underlying psycho-social and neurotic illness) is suddenly apparent to both doctor and patient
- Acts as a central point for change
- Consultation can now deal with the underlying basic 'Fault'

The Consultation

TATE'S TASKS
'THE DOCTORS COMMUNICATION HANDBOOK'

Involves use of concepts featured in other models. Similar to those used to assess tasks in the summative assessment and MRCGP videos.

1. Discover the reasons for attendance
- Listen to the patient's description of the symptom
- Obtain relevant social and occupational information
- Explore the patient's health understanding
- Enquire about other problems
- Obtain additional information about critical symptoms or other details
- Appropriate physical examination
- Make a working diagnosis

2. Define the clinical problem(s)

3. Address the patient's problems(s)
- Assess the severity of the presenting problem
- Choose an appropriate form of management
- Involve the patient in the management plan to the appropriate extent

4. Explain the problem(s) to the patient
- Share your findings with the patient
- Tailor the explanation to the needs of the patient
- Ensure that the explanation is understood and accepted by the patient

5. Make effective use of the consultation
- Make efficient use of resources – time, investigations, other professionals, etc.
- Establish an effective relationship with the patient

GLOSSARY

ACE	Angiotensin converting enzyme
ACEI	Angiotensin converting enzyme inhibitors
AD	Alzheimer's disease
AF	Atrial fibrillation
AOM	Acute otitis media
BHS	British hypertension society
BMA	British Medical Association
BMD	Bone mineral density
BMI	Body mass index
CBT	Cognitive behavoural therapy
CG	Clinical Governance
CHD	Coronary heart disease
CHI	Commission for health improvement
CME	Continued Medical Education
COAD	Chronic obstructive airways disease
COCP	Combined oral contraceptive pill
CPD	Continuous Professional Development
CPR	Cardiopulmonary resuscitation
CVD	Cardiovascular disease
DBP	Diastolic blood pressure
DEXA	Dual energy X-ray absorptiometry
DNR	Do not resuscitate
DSPD	Dangerous and severely personality disordered
DVLA	Driving vehicle licensing authority
DVT	Deep vein thrombosis
GI	Gastrointestinal
GMC	General Medical Council
GMS	General Medical Services
GPC	General Practitioners Committee
HA	Health Authority
HON	Health on the Net
HOT	Hypertension optimal treatment trial
HRT	Hormone replacement therapy
IHD	Ischaemic heart disease
ILA	Individual Learning Account
INR	International normalised ratio
LSPs	Local strategic partnerships
LVF	Left ventricular failure
MDU	Medical Defence Union
MI	Myocardial infarction

Glossary

MMR vaccine	Measles mumps rubella vaccine
NeLH	National Electronic Library for Health
NICE	National institute for clinical excellence
NNT	Number needed to treat
NRT	Nicotine replacement therapy
NSF	National service framework
OGTT	Oral glucose tolerance test
PCECs	Primary Care Emergency Centres
PCG	Primary Care Group
PCTs	Primary Care Trusts
PDPs	Personal Development Plans
PGEA	Postgraduate education allowance
PHCT	Primary Healthcare Trust
PMS	Personal Medical Services
PPDPs	Practice Professional Development Plans
PSA	Prostate specific antigen
RCP	Royal College of Physicians
RCT	Randomised controlled trial
SBP	Systolic blood pressure
SERMs	Selective oestrogen receptor modulators
SIDS	Sudden infant death syndrome
SSRIs	Selective serotonin reuptake inhibitors
STD	Sexually transmitted disease
TCA	Tricyclic antidepressant
TIA	Transient ischaemic attacks
tPA	Tissue plasminogen activator
URTI	Upper respiratory tract infection
WHO	World Health Organisation

JOURNALS REFERENCED
IN THIS BOOK

Ann Rheum Dis	Annals of the Rheumatic Diseases
Arch Dis Child	Archives of Diseases of Childhood
Arch Neuro	Archives of Neurology
BJGP	British Journal of General Practice
BMJ	British Medical Journal
Cerebrovasc Dis	Cerebrovascular Disorders
Circulation	Circulation
Clin Drug Invest	Clinical Drug Investigations
Diabetes	Diabetes
DTB	Drugs and Therapeutics Bulletin
Heart	Heart
JAMA	Journal of the American Medical Association
J Card Fail	Journal of Cardiac Failure
J consult Clin Psychol	Journal of Consulting and Clinical Psychology
J R Coll Gen Pract	Journal of the Royal College of General Practitioners
Lancet	The Lancet
NEMJ	New England Medical Journal
Osteoporosis Review	Osteoporosis Review
Thorax	Thorax

INDEX

Acute otitis media 123–125
   antibiotics
Advance directives 195
Age discrimination 78
Alcohol 68–69
Alternative medicine 180–182
Angiotensin
   II receptor antagonists 14
   converting enzyme
      inhibitors 13
Anorexia nervosa 66
Antibiotic resistance 122
Asthma 32–34
   self-management 33
Atrial fibrillation 16–18
   risk of stroke 18

Beta-blockers 14
Bisphosphonates 29
Bulimia nervosa 66
Bupropion 37

Calcium 30
Cancer 114–121
   NHS Plan 114
   prostate 119–121
   screening 116
Cannabis 71
Cardiovascular trials 7, 9, 15
Chlamydia 106–107
Cholesterol
   lowering 6
Chronic obstructive airways
   disease 35
Clinical
   governance 129–134
   guidelines 192–194
Confidentiality 186

Consent 188
Consultation 208–219
   models 213–219
Contraception
   emergency 100–102
Coronary heart disease 5–10
   guidelines 6
   risk factors 6
Counselling 72–73

Data Protection Act 187
Deep vein thrombosis 97
Dementia 88, 93–96
Depression 56–61, 87
   drugs 58
   post-natal 62
   St John's Wort 61, 181
Diabetes control and
   complications trial 24
Diabetes mellitus 22–27
   cardiovascular disease 25
   diagnosis 22
   drugs 26
   hypertension 25
   screening programme 25
   studies 24
DiClemente and Proschaska's
   cycle of change 39
Digoxin 14
Diuretics 13
Doctor-patient partnership 212
Drugs 70–71
   anti-psychotic 64–65

Eating disorders 66–67
Elderly 74
   dementia 88, 93
   depression 87

223

Index

general hospital care 81
health care 75
intermediate care 81
mental health 86
osteoporosis 86
person-centred care 79
society 76
End of life decisions 196–200
Ethics 205–207
European stroke initiative 19

Falls 84
Framingham data 2

General Medical Council 183
complaints 184
General Practice
computer-generated
repeat perscriptions 174
funding 156
future 146
NHS Plan 147
out of hours care and
24 hour responsibility 163
Gingko biloba 181

Heart failure 13–15
High risk patients 53
Homeopathy 182
Hormone replacement
therapy 30, 108–110
Hypertension 1–4
BHS risk tables 2, 3
investigations 4
optimal treatment trial 1
society guidelines 1

Influenza 42–44
vaccine 42
Inhalers 32

Learning portfolio 144
Levonelle-2 101

Medicine and Internet 177–179
Medico-legal issues and
guidelines 183-191
confidentiality 186
consent 188
Mental health act
reform 49

National Service Framework
coronary heart
disease 10–12
mental health 48–55
Negligence 190
NHS
Direct 153, 165-166
Net 178
Plan 147
cancer 114
General Practice 147–157
NICE guidelines
asthma 32
Nicotine replacement therapy 37
Nurse Practitioners 168–171

Obesity 45–47
Obstructive airways disease,
chronic 35
Oral contraceptive pill 97–99
benefits 99
risks 98
Orlistat 45

Index

Osteoporosis 28–31
    cortico-steroid induced 28
    drugs 29
      bisphosphonates
    identification of high
      risk patients 28
Out of hours care 163
Outreach clinics 172

Personal medical services 161
Practice
    formulary 173
    personal development
      plans 141
    professional
      development plans 143
Prescriptions,
    computer-generated 174
Primary Care Groups 154, 160
Prostate cancer 119
PSA levels 119
Psychiatry
    anti-psychotic drugs 64
    counselling 72

RALES study 14
Ramipril 8
Rationing 158–159
Reductil 46
Refugees 201–204
Relenza 42
Revalidation 135–145
    practice and personal
      development plans 141

Schizophrenia 63
SCOFF questionnaire 67
Selective oestrogen receptor
    modulator therapy 30

Self-regulation 135
Shipman case 175
Smoking cessation 36–41
    guidelines 36
Sore throat 126–128
Spironolactone 14
St John's wort 61, 181
Statins 31
STORM 46
Stroke 19–21, 82
    interventions 20–21
    national service
      framework 20
Sudden infant death
    syndrome 113

Teenagers
    contraception 105
    pregnancy 104
    sexual health 103–105

UK prospective diabetes
    study 24

Vaccinations 111–112
    influenza 42
    meningococcal C 111
    MMR 111
Vitamin D 30

Walk-in centres 167
Warfarin 15
Wilson's criteria for
    screening 116

Zyban 37

225

PASTEST REVISION BOOKS

MRCGP Practice Papers: MCQs and EMQs Second Edition
P Ellis and P Elliott   *1 901198 29 4*
- Five complete MCQ and EMQ Practice Papers
- Correct answers and detailed teaching notes
- Expert advice on successful exam technique
- Comprehensive Revision Index for easy reference to specific topics
- Invaluable intensive practice material for all MRCGP candidates

MRCGP: Approaching the New Modular Examination
J Sandars   *0 906896 64 9*
- Written specifically for the modular exam format
- Compiled by a current Royal College examiner, this book covers all components of the new exam
- 100 MCQs with correct answers and teaching notes
- Eight Critical Appraisal questions based on recent BMJ articles
- Tips on tackling the Audit section

Practice Papers for the DCH Examination
J Lynch   *1 901198 52 9*
- Three complete practice papers
- 180 MCQs, 30 Short Note questions and 6 case commentaries
- Section on tackling the Clinical Components
- Comprehensive MCQ Revision Index

DRCOG Practice Exams: MCQs and OSCEs
M Dooley   *0 906896 44 4*
- Two complete MCQ Practice Exams with correct answers and detailed teaching notes
- Twenty OSCE questions with model answers
- Written by two Royal College examiners
- Invaluable Revision Checklist covering the complete syllabus
- Expert advice on exam technique

To Order: For 24 hour order despatch call 01565 752000 or shop at www.pastest.co.uk

PASTEST REVISION COURSES

MRCGP

All PasTest MRCGP courses, including Hot Topics Days, are PGEA Approved

Dynamic and knowledgeable lecturers
Most of our lecturers are Royal College examiners, providing you with the ultimate advantage. With many years membership experience, the tutors have intimate knowledge of the exam and adjust their teaching to reflect the current trends. Throughout the course, they provide valuable tips about exam technique. We constantly evaluate our lecturers through feedback from candidates to ensure that our courses are continually improved.

Impressive pre-course material
Exclusive course notes are provided, including a complete set of Paper 1 and Paper 2 questions, with diagrams, lists, mnemonics and revision checklists. During the course you will receive correct answers and teaching notes, written by our team of MRCGP question writers.

Course content 100% relevant to the exam
All our MRCGP courses consist of modular sessions, which provide intensive practice of the key elements of the exam. The course is designed to mirror the modular format of the MRCGP EXAMINATION.

The course content includes sessions dedicated to Papers 1 and 2, where you will receive model answers and detailed feedback on the extensive pre-course material. In addition, our tutors will provide invaluable advice on the topics that are likely to appear in the current exam as well as hints and tips on exam technique.

To prepare you for the Oral examination, the College Examiners will provide an insight into what the examiners are looking for. You will then be divided into small groups to practise your technique. You will also receive expert advice, hints and tips on consultation skills to ensure you receive the most complete preparation.

PasTest Revision Courses

New: Hot Topics Day

In response to persistent demand from customers, we have introduced a new Hot Topics Day. Rather than just enabling you to quote a list of references, the Hot Topics Day is intended to provide a solid foundation for revision by providing you with a thorough understanding of the relevant study topics. Teaching sessions and comprehensive handouts on the day will cover a wide spectrum of subject areas.

In addition to clinical subjects, the day will focus on new developments in General Practice, including revalidation, clinical governance and personal development plans. As a result of the recent changes in the MRCGP examination, it is essential that you have a working knowledge of Hot Topics. This course will not only provide you with an invaluable advantage when you take your exam, but will also be of great benefit in your future career in General Practice.

Consolidate your learning with a PasTest revision course, call now for details:

01565 752000

BOOK ONLINE AT www.pastest.co.uk